Looking Good to Feel Good

Stories of Breast Cancer, Breast Reconstruction, Bravery and Happiness

Photography and Design by Scott Walz
Introduction and Pearls by Sandra Bouzaglou, MD, FACS

Hello Gorgeous Publishing

Contributors:

Book Designer: Scott Walz, Sandra Bouzaglou, MD,FACS

Photography: Scott Walz, Studio Walz, Inc. www.studiowalz.com

Introduction, Pearls: Sandra Bouzaglou, MD,FACS

Stories written by: The Survivors themselves

Story Editor: Cynthia Ellingsen

Scarves: Paige Hoogerheide, PA

Breast Reconstruction Awareness Logo: Daniel J. Archer

www.center4plasticsurgery.com

Intro

One out of every eight women in the United States will develop breast cancer in her lifetime. There are over 2.5 million women in the United States who are breast cancer survivors and—due to improved methods for early diagnosis, improved therapies, and gene testing—more women are surviving this devastating disease.[1] Years ago, women diagnosed with breast cancer underwent radical mastectomies with disfiguring results, leaving them with caved-in chests and swollen arms.

More recently, breast conservation therapy (or lumpectomy) offered women the ability to keep their breasts; however, a large percentage of them were still unhappy with their cosmetic results and eventually sought further reconstructive surgery.[2] For those who underwent radiation therapy as well as lumpectomy, attempts at reconstruction brought a much higher risk of complications and often required "flaps" from another part of the body to rebuild the breast.

Mastectomy and lumpectomy both continue to offer a chance for a cure and, if therapy is properly coordinated between the cancer surgeon and the plastic surgeon, then immediate reconstruction can offer the best cosmetic result. In fact, breast incisions designed by a plastic surgeon can give an aesthetic result that looks just like a cosmetic breast lift or breast reduction. The women in this book will exemplify this.

With the advent of genetic testing for BRCA1 and BRCA2, the number of women requesting prophylactic mastectomy is increasing, despite the fact that BRCA accounts for only 5 to 10 percent of all breast cancers.[3] Angelina Jolie bravely underwent

Sandra Bouzaglou, MD FACS

"Because when you look good you feel good"

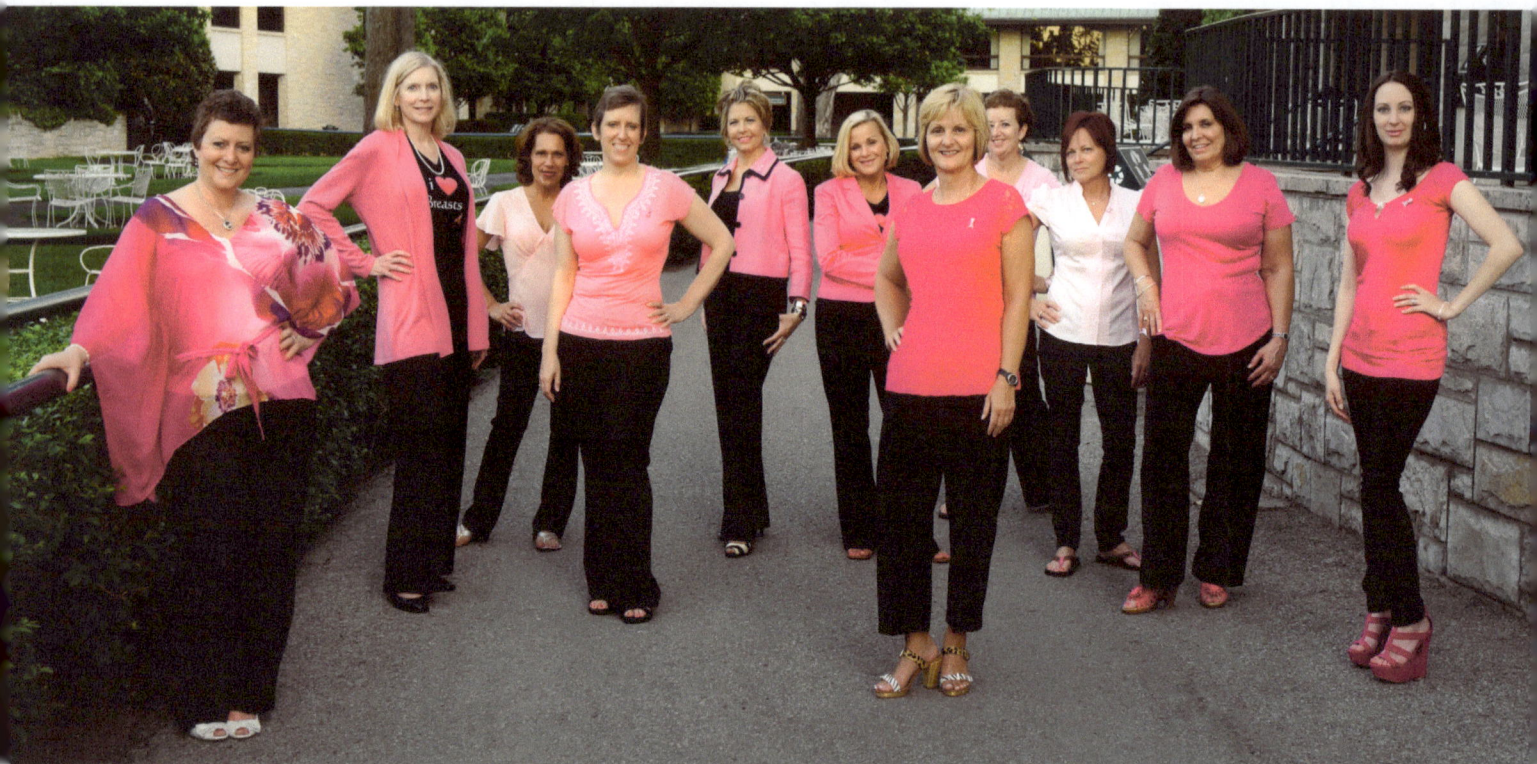

a double mastectomy with immediate reconstruction and shared her story publicly. This should help to erase some of the stigma associated with the diagnosis of breast cancer. Through her story, perhaps more women will not be afraid to act proactively, obtain early mammograms, seek medical attention when a lump is felt, or undergo gene testing if they have a strong positive family history of breast cancer.

Of all American women who undergo mastectomy, a minority of women choose reconstruction.[4] Why? Well, there are many reasons. Women diagnosed with breast cancer are often initially overwhelmed by the diagnosis and seek to have the cancer removed as quickly as possible without attempting to think about how they will look or feel after surgery. A surgical oncologist who may mention breast reconstruction or perhaps provide reading material about reconstruction first sees them; however, a consultation with a plastic surgeon is not part of their standard treatment plan. These women, unfortunately, are uninformed of all of their options. Other reasons include diagnosis at an advanced stage where surgery is not an initial option. Geographical location, varying socioeconomic and racial ethnic minority groups, has also been shown to influence whether a patient chooses breast reconstruction or not. [4,6]

Many women think that breast reconstruction is a cosmetic procedure not covered by their insurance, and thus think they cannot afford it. Thanks to the Women's Health and Cancer Rights Act signed into law by President Bill Clinton in 1998, health insurers in the United States are required to cover the cost of breast reconstruction and any symmetrical procedures of the opposite side. Despite this, less than one out of five women who undergo mastectomy go on to have breast reconstruction.

More recently, a bill known as known as the "Breast Cancer Patient Education Act of 2013"[9] was introduced in Congress in May 2013. This act is meant to implement an educational campaign to inform breast cancer patients needing surgery regarding the availability of coverage of breast reconstruction, prostheses, and other options, with a focus of informing patients who are members of racial and ethnic minority groups. Hopefully, this new act will empower all women diagnosed with breast cancer to understand the treatment options that will best meet their personal needs.

As a board-certified plastic surgeon with more than twenty years of experience, I have seen an increasing number of women diagnosed with breast cancer. The majority of my practice involves breast reduction for symptoms such as back pain, shoulder pain, etc. Despite negative preoperative mammograms, however, we have also diagnosed numerous breast cancers in breast reduction

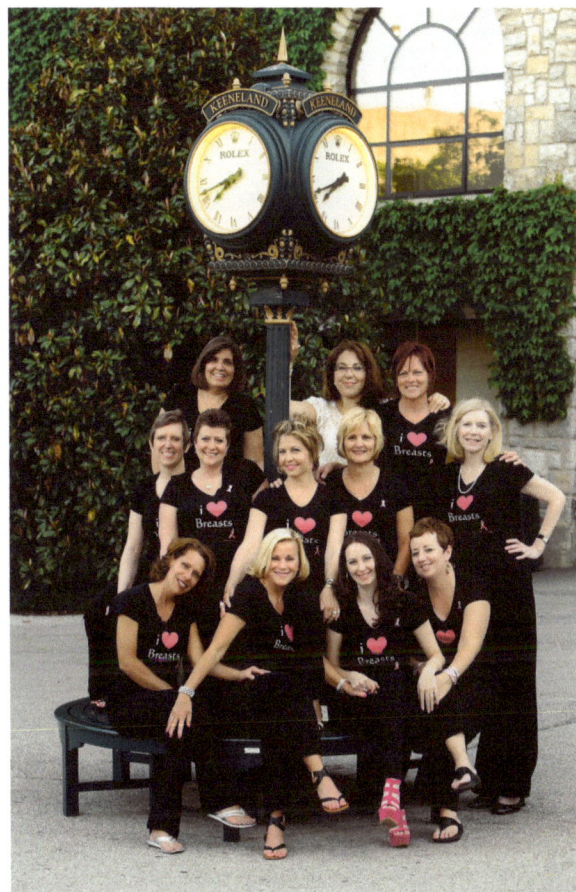

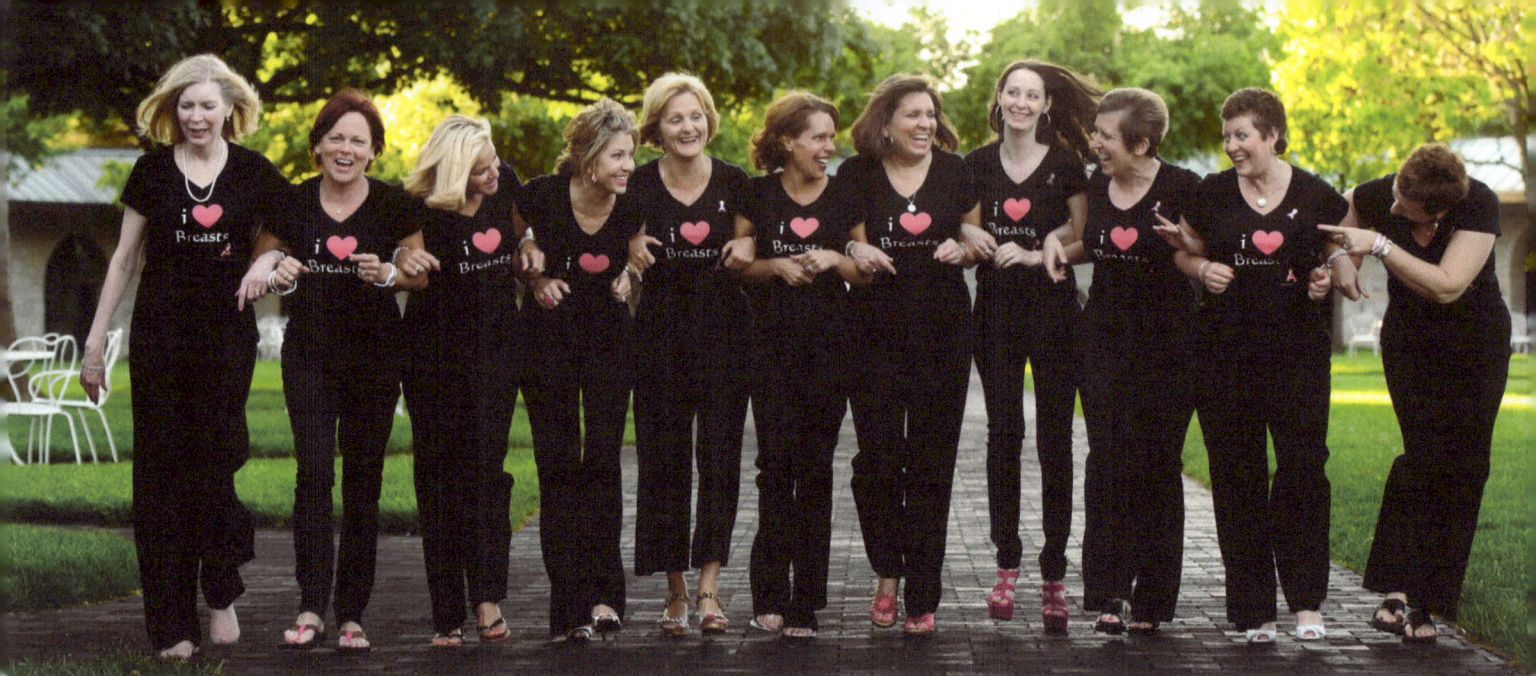

specimens. Fortunately, these were all early cancers that could not have been detected by today's methods. Some of these patients opted to have chemotherapy and no further surgery, but many went on to have complete mastectomies and immediate implant reconstruction using the breast reduction incisions. Their final cosmetic result was no different than if they had had a simple breast reduction. That led me to think—why are we not designing mastectomy or even lumpectomy incisions from the very beginning?

This book was written, along with these inspiring ladies, to help raise awareness of the positive effects that immediate breast reconstruction can have on women who are diagnosed with breast cancer. In the pages that follow, thirteen brave women from various walks of life—my patients from around the beautiful state of Kentucky—proudly discuss and display the results of their breast reconstruction procedures. Together we hope that we can inspire breast cancer patients to know all of their options and make an informed decision from the time they are diagnosed with breast cancer.

Italian surgeon and father of plastic surgery, Dr. Guspar Tagliacozzi, in 1597, stated "*We restore, repair, and make whole parts…which nature has given but which fortune has taken away, not so much that they may delight the eye, but that they buoy up the spirit and help the mind of the afflicted."* My goal in breast reconstruction is to allow the patient to look and feel like a centerfold once their procedure is complete. I want them to look good, not only in clothing but without, as well. Because when you look good, you feel good!

The women whose stories you will read in the following pages have experienced just that. In fact, not only were their spirits lifted, but mine were lifted as well. They have shown me that all of my years of training—from UCLA, to medical school in Chicago, through five years of general surgery at The University of Iowa, and finally to plastic surgery training at the University of Kentucky— have given me a purpose for what I do. The most rewarding part of this project came when I accompanied our wonderful photographer, Scott Walz, to interview and photograph these amazing women in their own hometowns. Getting to know the families and friends who care for them helped me understand how important plastic surgery is and how proud I am to have made a positive difference in their lives. Enjoy and be ready to put a smile on your face and say WOW!

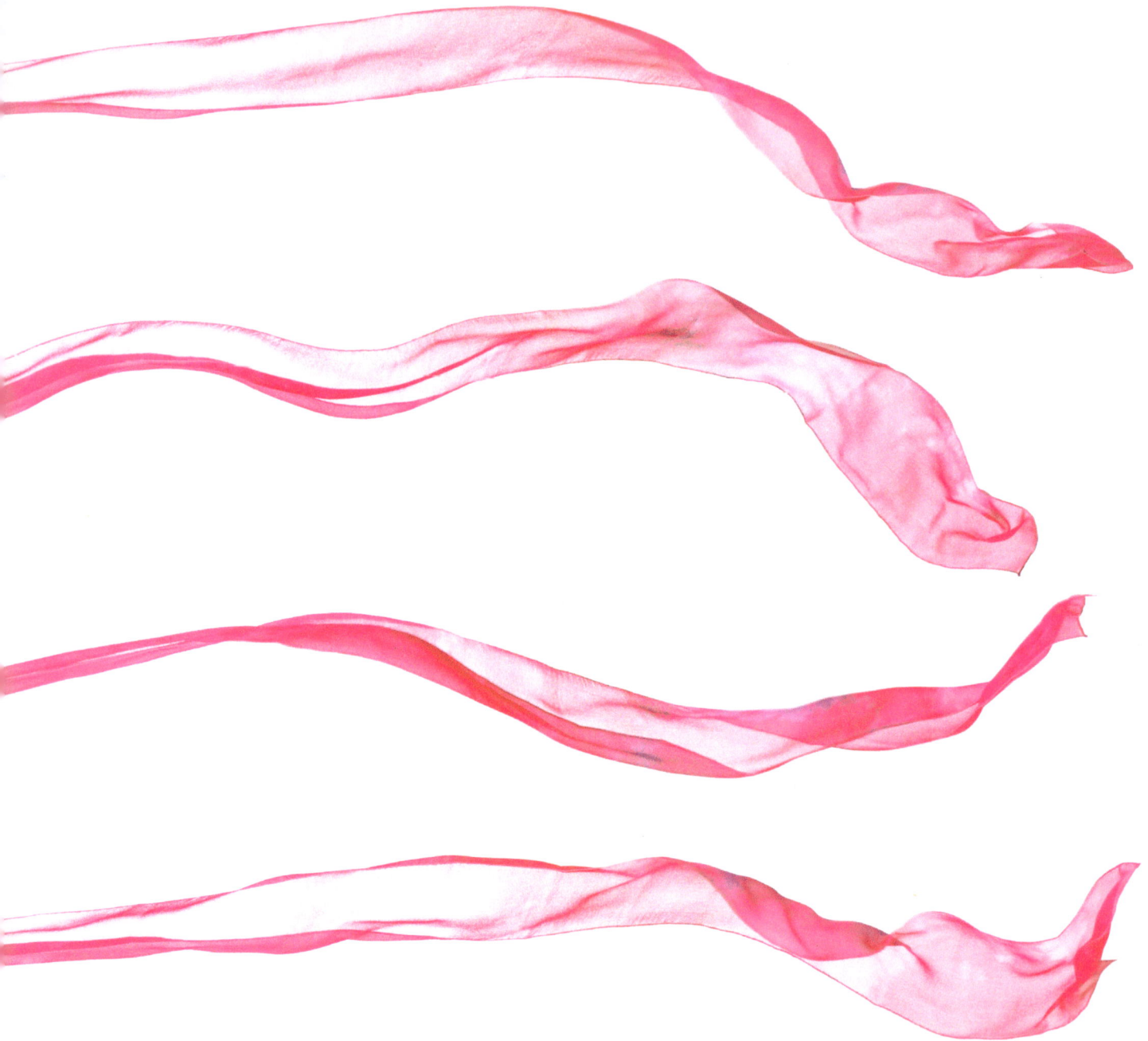

Their Stories

Genea
Alycia
Sandy
Sherry
Beverly
Jill
Mary
Lisa
Susan
Lisa
Shawna
Marsha
Holly

Edited by Cynthia Ellingsen

Genea

My name is Genea and I have been fighting Breast Cancer since October 26, 2011.

I was forty-five years old when diagnosed with Invasive Ductal Carcinoma. I had my bi-lateral mastectomy on November 18, 2011. During my surgery, it was confirmed that the cancer had spread to my lymph nodes. I started chemo on December 26, 2011.

I am a mother of two wonderful young men and a wife to a very loyal husband. Being the one that "was never sick", I knew it would be devastating to some of my friends and family to learn that I had breast cancer. I had protected and sheltered my boys their entire lives; now, I was about to turn their world upside down.

I knew how sickened they would feel – years before, I had been on their end of the conversation when my mother told me she had Ovarian Cancer. Sadly, she lost her battle just eight months after her diagnosis. I was twenty-six at the time and my

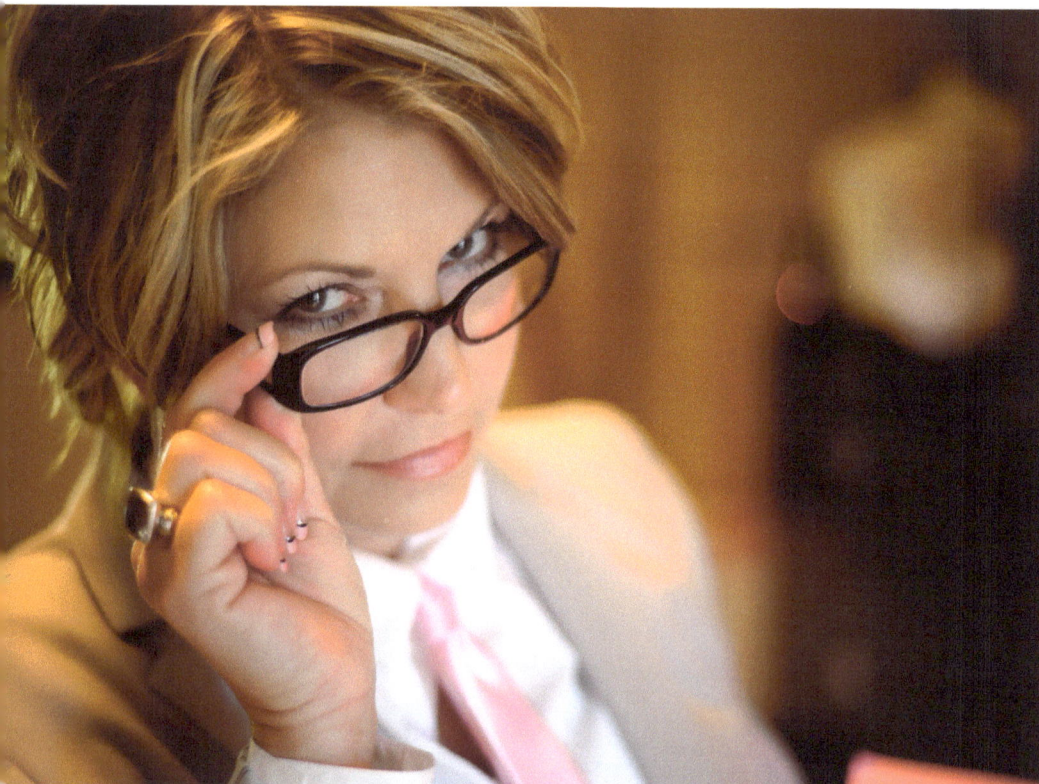

first-born son was just eleven months old. I had to be strong then to take care of my baby and have "no fear".

After seeing the fear in the eyes of my loved ones, I made a decision to have "no fear" once again. It was an easy decision to make. I have always put others before myself and this time, I had no choice but to be strong. I had to think about my boys, family and close friends; if I chose to be in good spirits, everyone else around me would be, as well.

My boys and many others remained at my side throughout every surgery, chemo, head shaving party, etc. My oldest son's fiancé was there for me as well. She is the daughter I never had. I reassured all of them that I would be just fine and that this was just temporary.

Once I received the news of my diagnosis, I did have to educate myself on many things. I did not know who my surgeon would be for the bi-lateral mastectomy. However, I knew who would do my reconstruction.

I had met her several years prior. I now call her my "reconstruction artist", as cancer took the "womanly" things from me such as my breast, hair and eyelashes; I knew that she would make

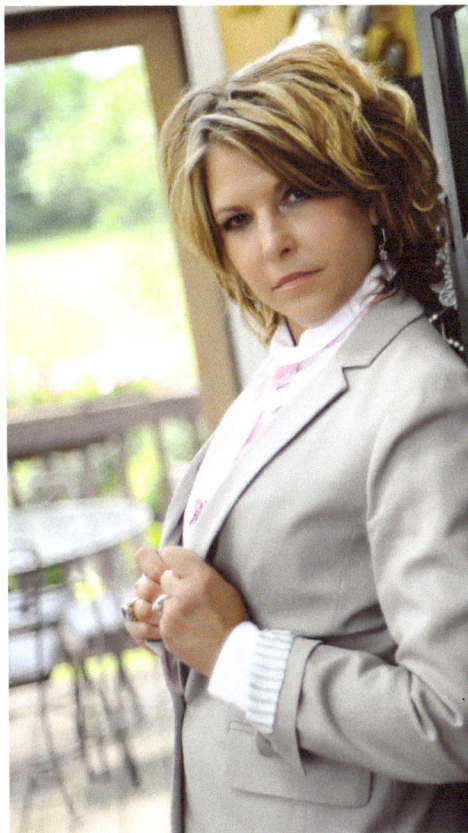

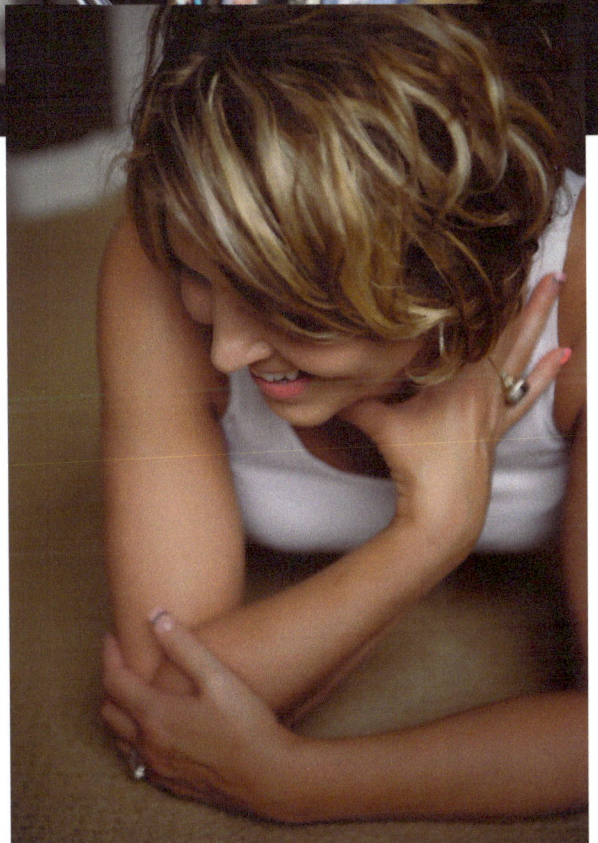

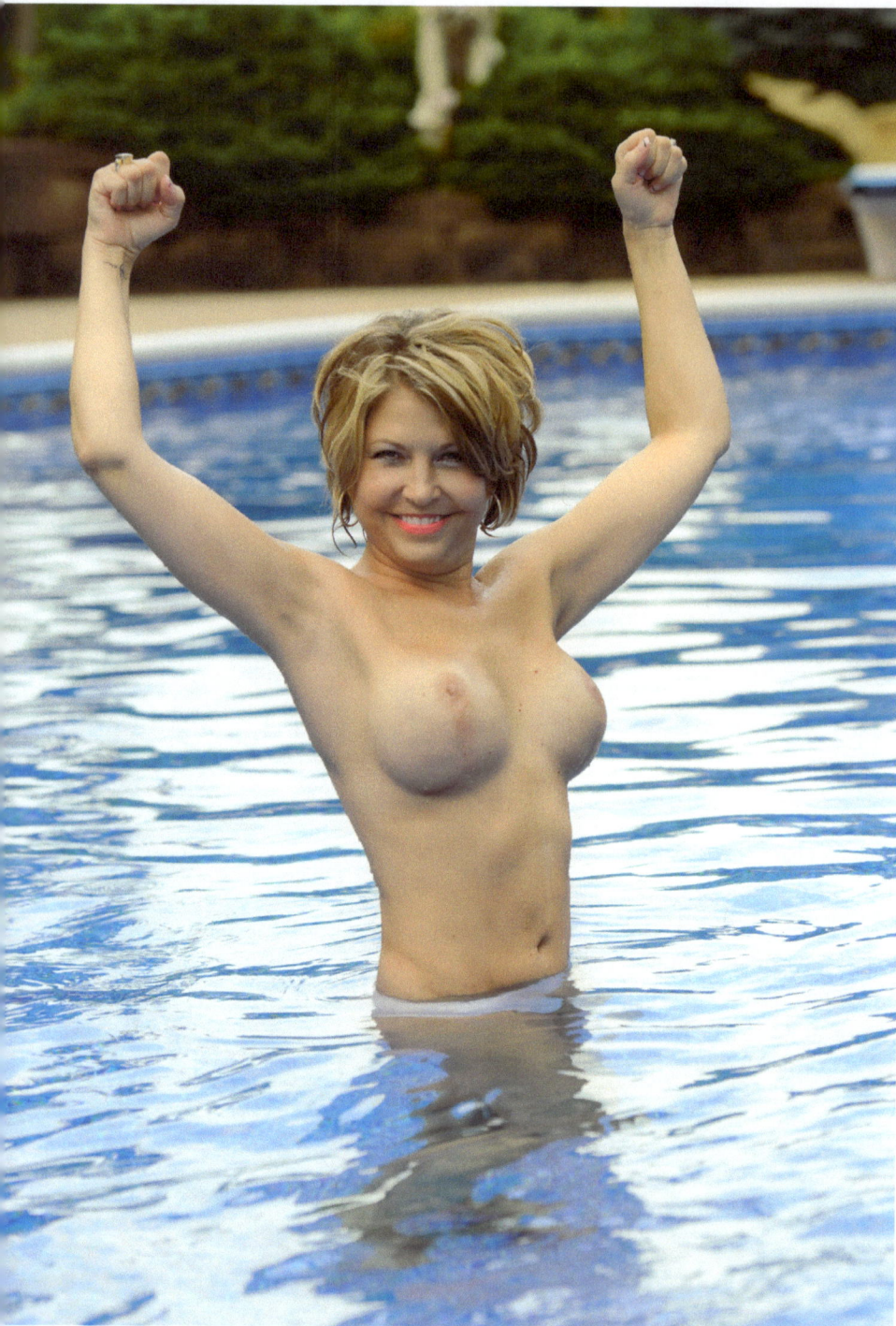

> *"I have a tattoo on my right inner wrist that says "no fear". It reminds me of my many battles including cancer and how I conquered them."*

me as whole as possible. Thanks to her work, I am still very much a woman.

To me and many other women, the option to lose your breasts to save your life makes all kinds of things run through your mind. You wonder how your body will look and if you will ever be the same. Well, I am not the same. How could I be, after all I have been through? Numerous surgeries, six months of chemo and hospitalizations…

But thanks to modern medicine, I am stronger and more beautiful than ever before. Mastectomy is such a frightening and sickening word but if you get a plastic surgeon involved from the very beginning, your end results can have a very positive impact on your life.

In my younger years, I was raised with an abusive alcoholic father. I learned very quickly to have "no fear", to be strong and that laughter could be my best friend. Over the years, I have had many struggles but they prepared me for my battle with Cancer. I call these "speed bumps" in LIFE!

12

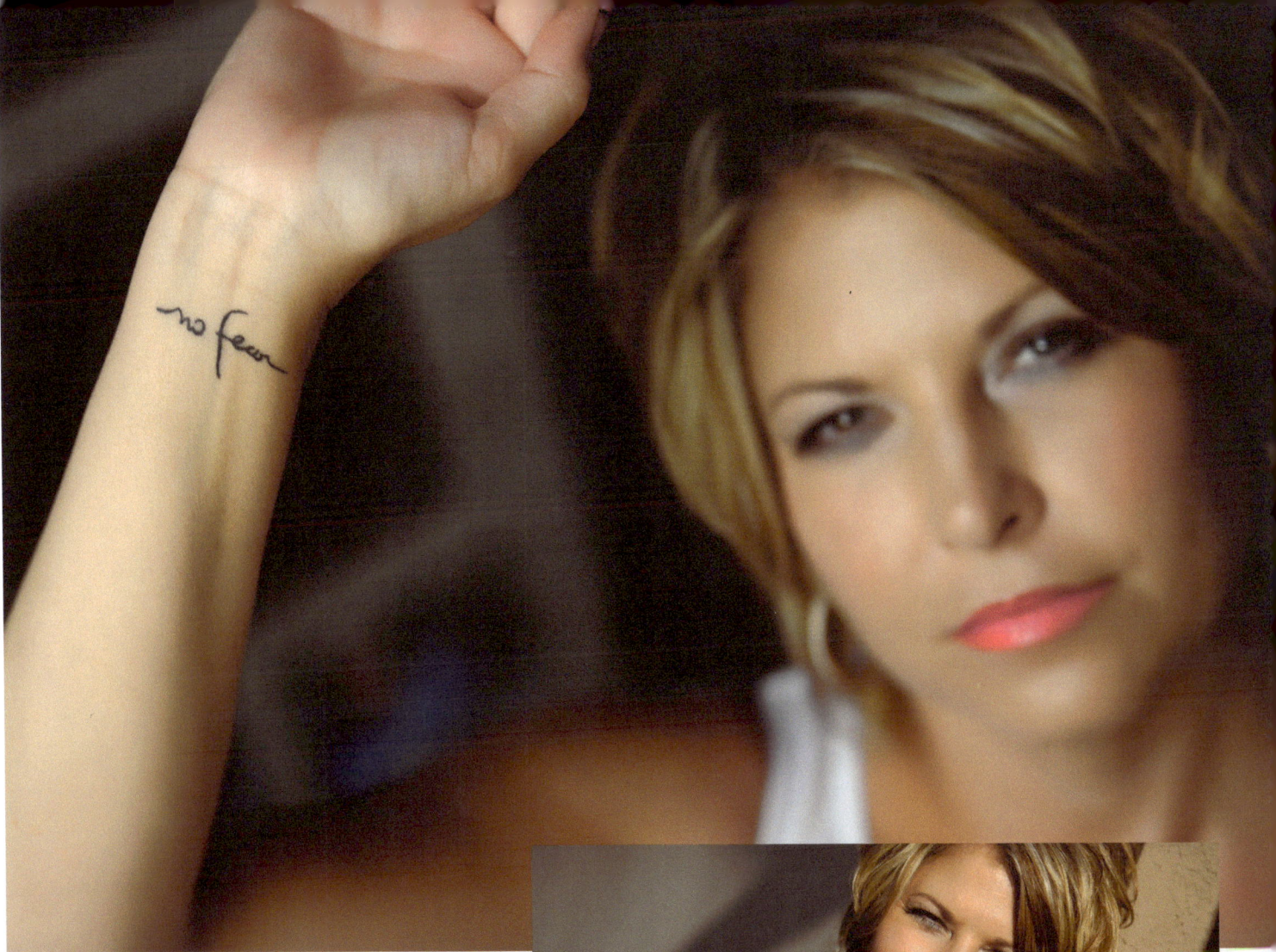

I have a tattoo on my right inner wrist that says "no fear". It reminds me of my many battles including cancer and how I conquered them. Cancer took enough from me - it could not take my spirit! We have no guarantee of to-morrow, anyway. Cancer just affirmed that for me.

Since my diagnosis, I have spent many hours reaching out to other women that have been

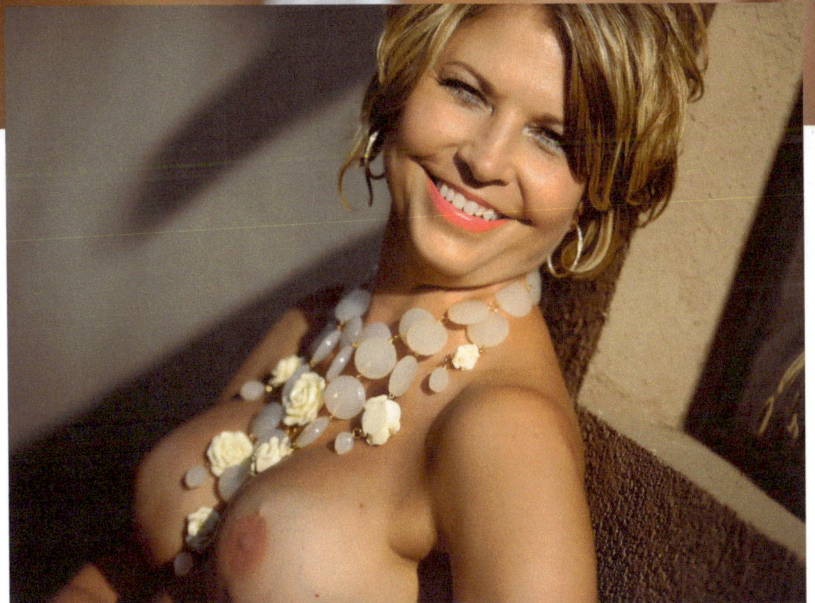

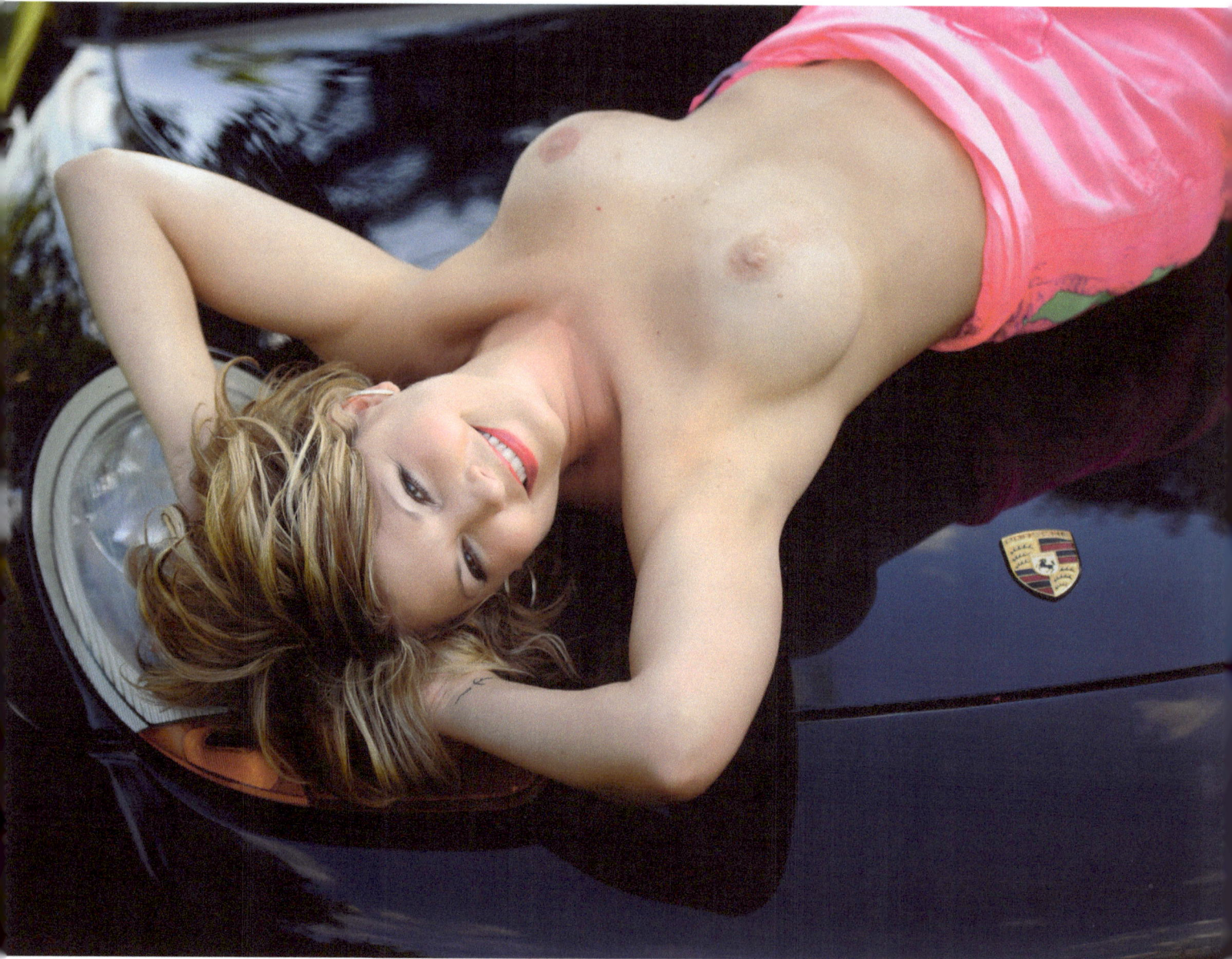

diagnosed with Breast Cancer. So many women are not made aware of all of their choices and that they need to get plastic surgery involved from the very beginning. Every woman is different and each diagnosis is different, but it is possible to have a positive outcome. I want to reassure them that they are not alone.

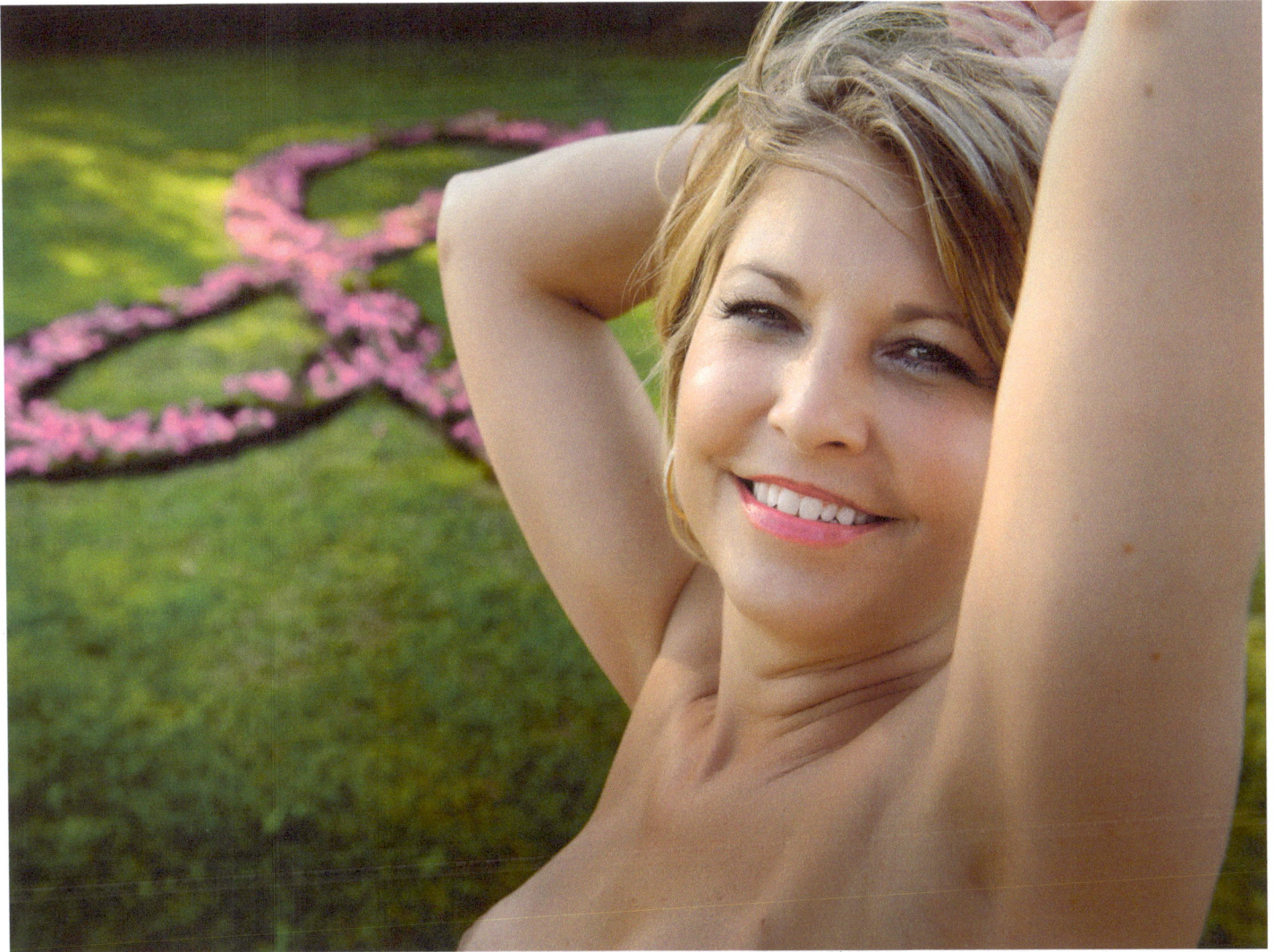

We hope this book helps you. I am very proud of my results and you can be too!

Genea
Breast Cancer Warrior

Alycia

What a great gift: I received cosmetic breast augmentation in October of 2009. It was an anniversary gift, to celebrate nine years with my husband. I went from a 34 A to a 34 B and they looked amazing!

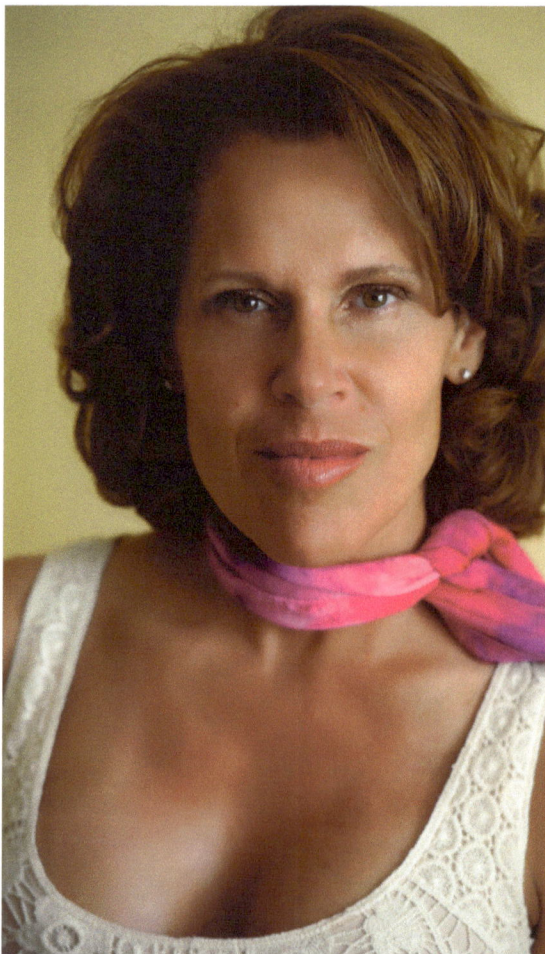

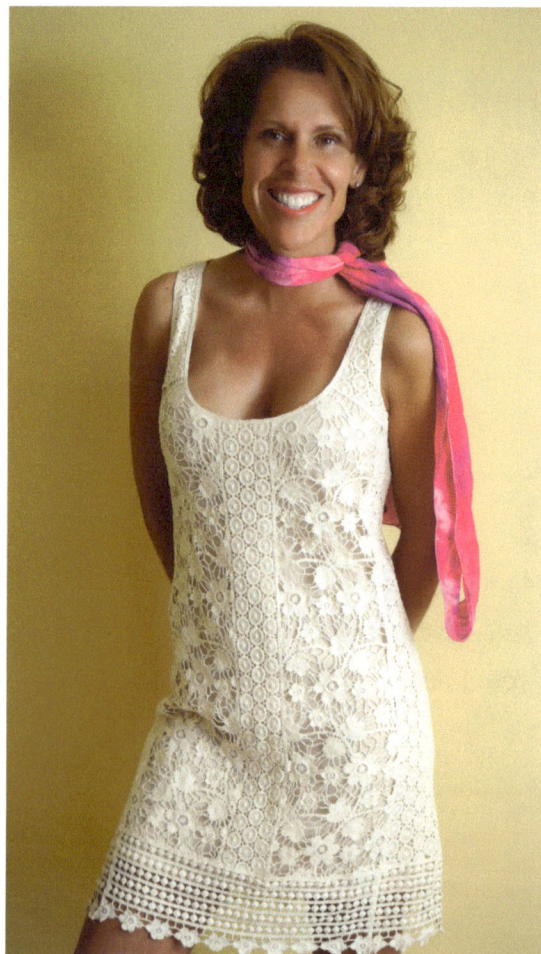

In May 2010, I went for my annual mammogram and it was normal. In June, I felt a small lump in my right breast. I have fibrocystic breasts, so I thought nothing of it but by the end of July, it had grown large enough that you could see it through a clingy t-shirt.

I went to my family practice doctor, who sent me to get an ultra sound and biopsy. The comments I kept hearing were reassuring: it must be something to do with my breast implants, it did not look like cancer...

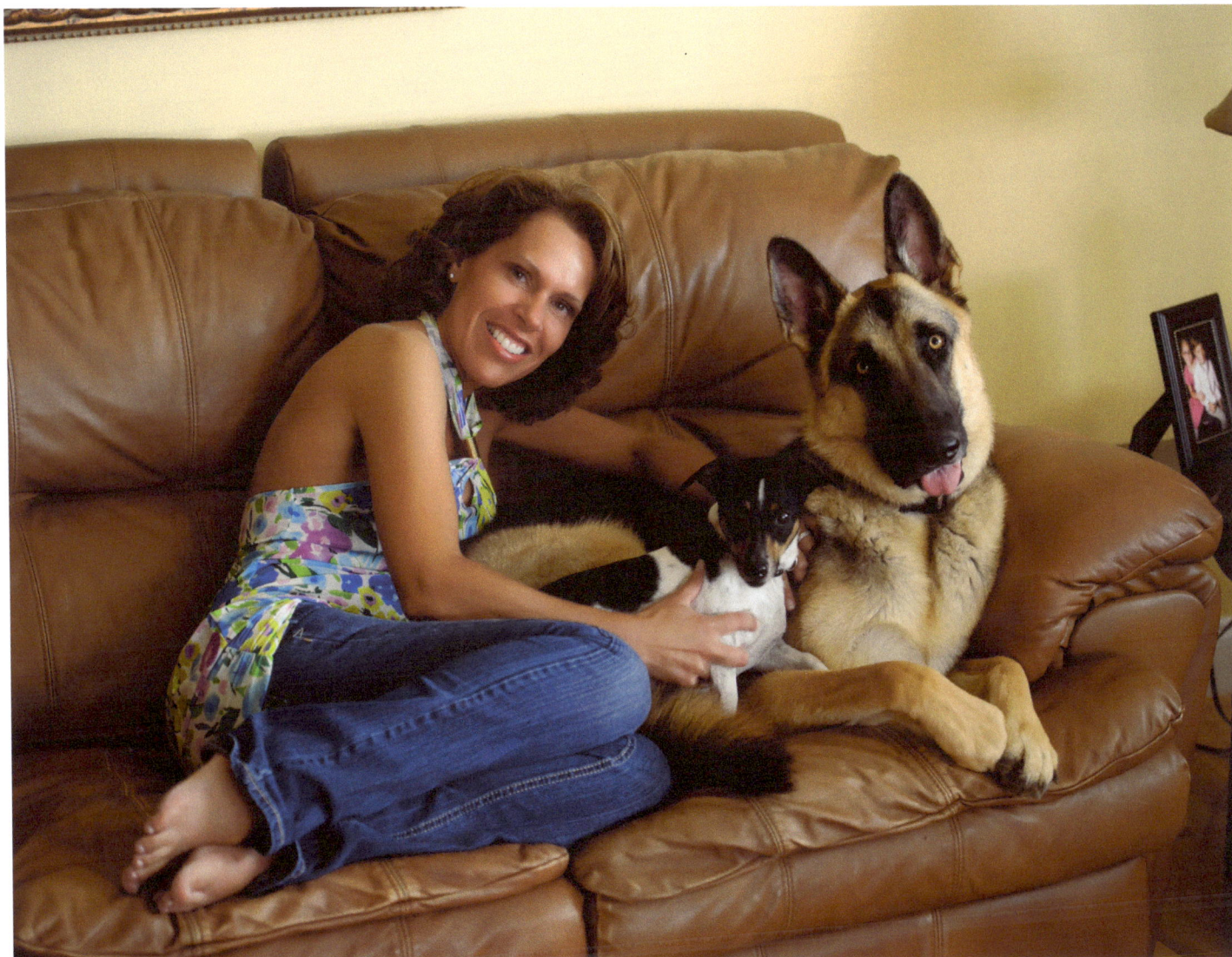

The radiologist did not want to do a needle biopsy, so I was set up for surgery to have the lump surgically removed just a few days after my first visit to my family Doctor.

I never thought about it. My surgery went well. The mass was removed.

That evening I received a devastating phone call: I had breast cancer. Stage 2-estrogen positive.

Five days later, I had a right-sided mastectomy with immediate re-

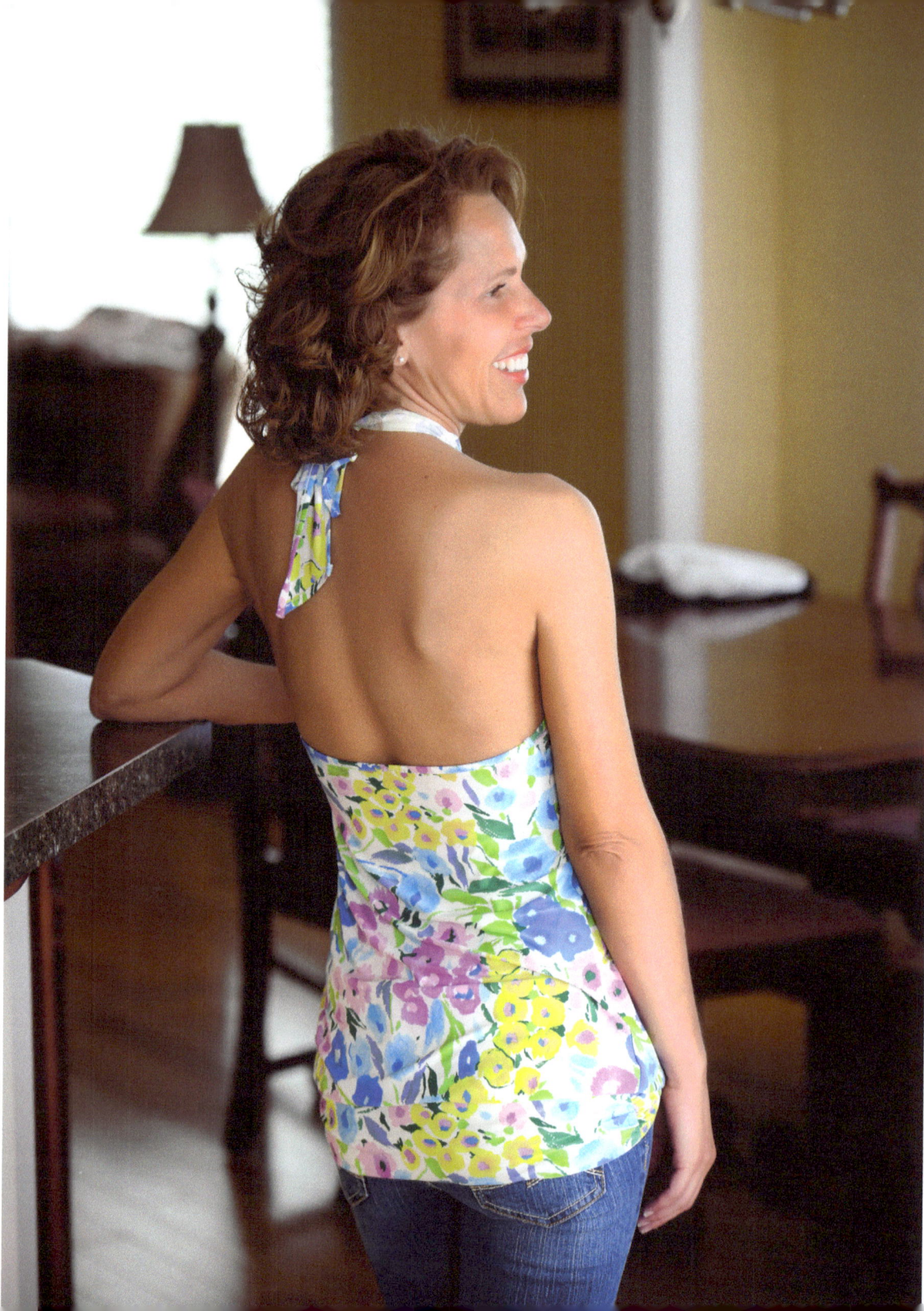

> ## "I believe that my breasts are a part of my womanly beauty, and I wanted them back!"

construction. From there, I underwent five months of chemotherapy. It took nine surgeries/procedures to reconstruct my breast(s) to their current state.

No woman should feel less than a woman because of breast cancer.

I believe that my breasts are a part of my womanly beauty, and I wanted them back! So, reconstructive surgery was always a must for me. No matter how many I had to go through, I needed to do it for myself. I would not let cancer take away my breasts.

I was diagnosed with breast cancer when I was thirty-nine. Now, I am forty-one. I fought through numerous surgeries and battled the pain both physically and emotionally with the help of my children, my love and my God to win this!

This journey has been

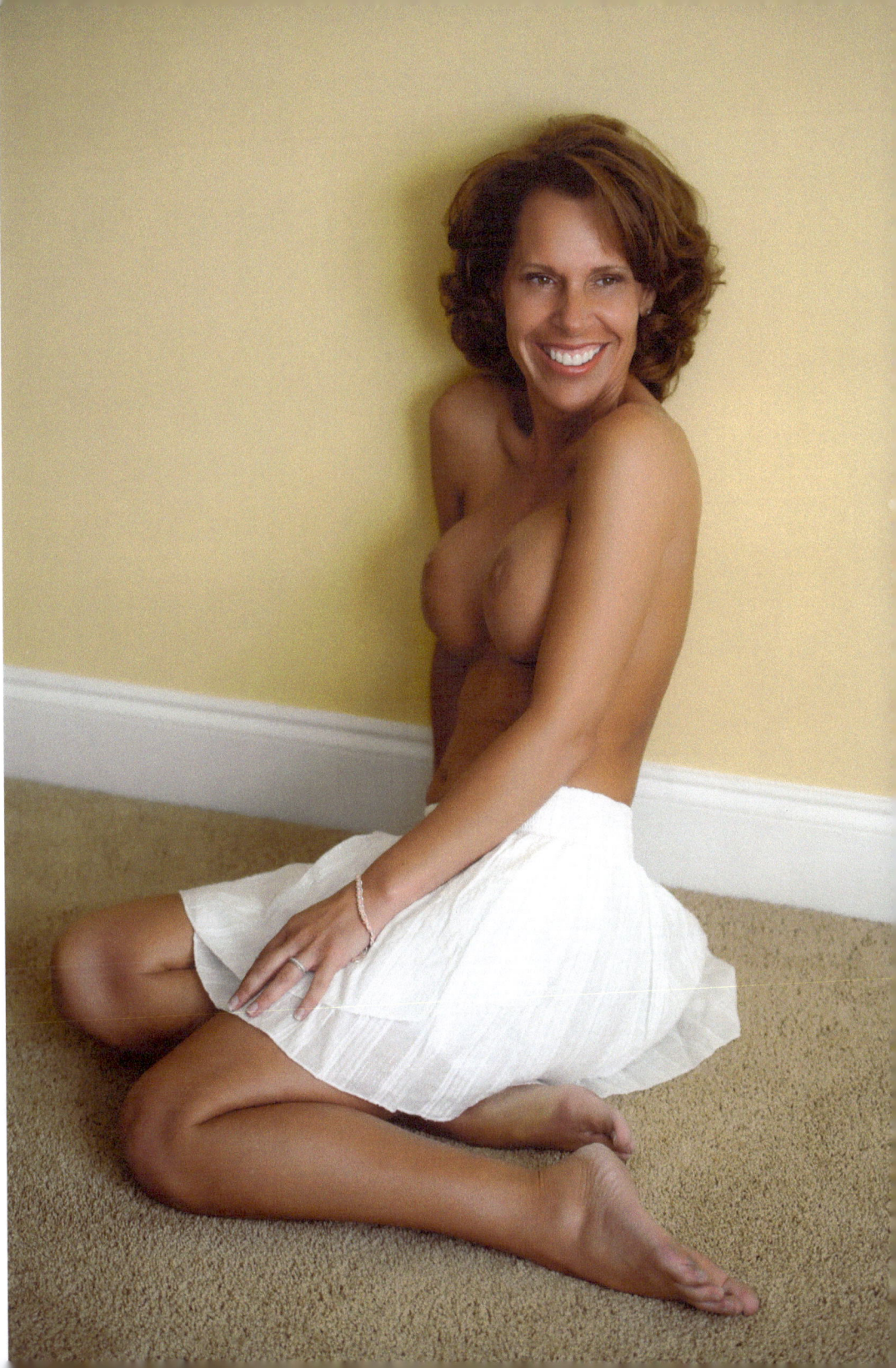

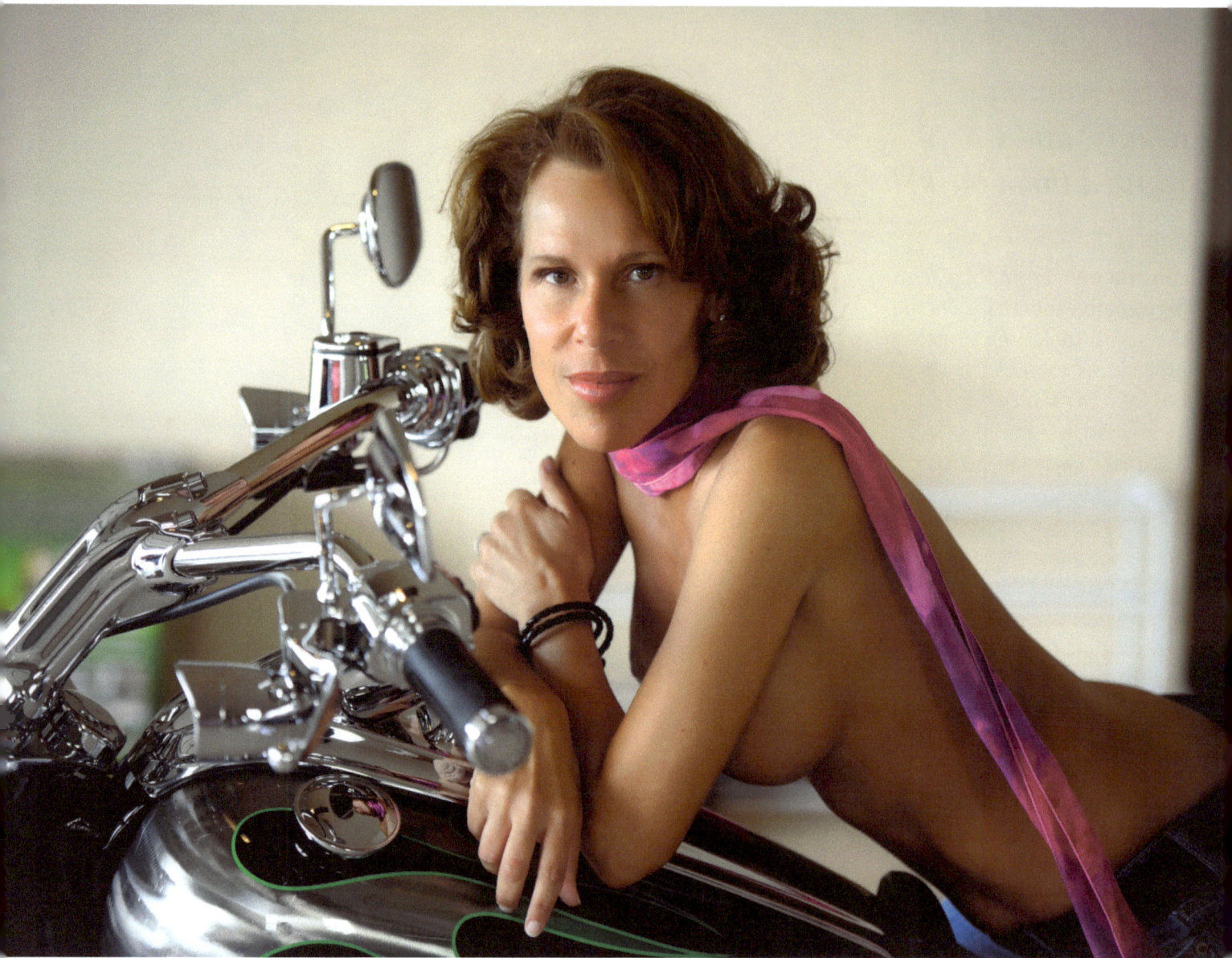

long and painful, but also very spiritually awakening. My personal relationship with Jesus Christ has been my strength throughout. I have also learned that both the survivor and the family who wear the pink ribbon must be strong throughout the fight.

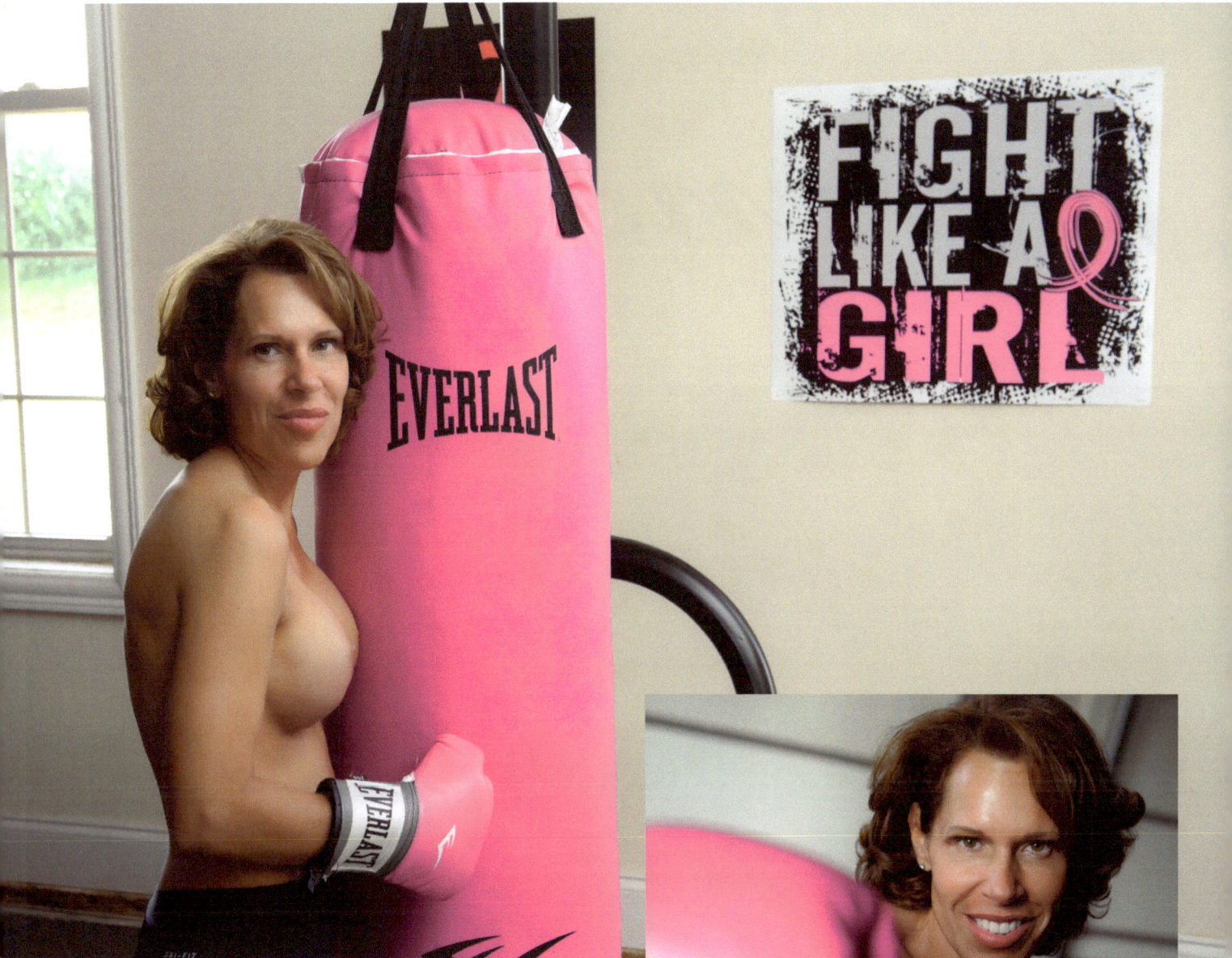

I wouldn't go through breast cancer again if I had a choice, but I was chosen, therefore I will continue to be a role model for all who have to battle breast cancer.

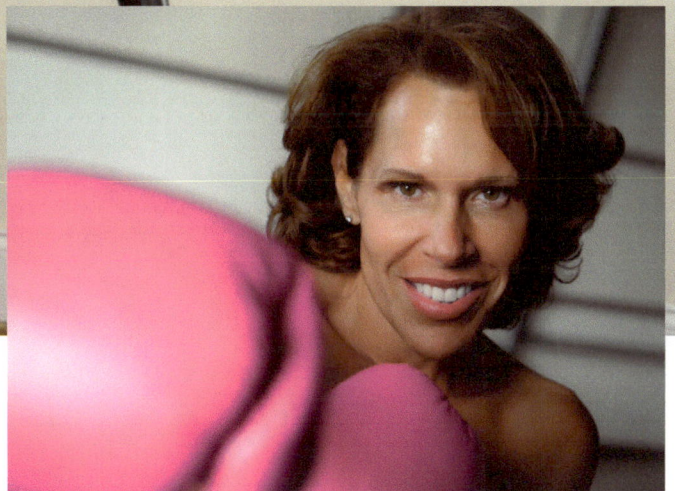

Sandy

I am currently fifty-four years old. My story begins on December 27th, 2011, when I received a call to come back for another mammogram right away. The timing for this phone call was not good, but it never is.

When the call came, I was at my dad's house arranging for hospice to come in and planning a trip to see my in-laws for the holidays. I was more concerned about my very ill father and what was happening with him. I was also busy raising my grandchild, as I had been since he was eleven months old, in addition to worrying

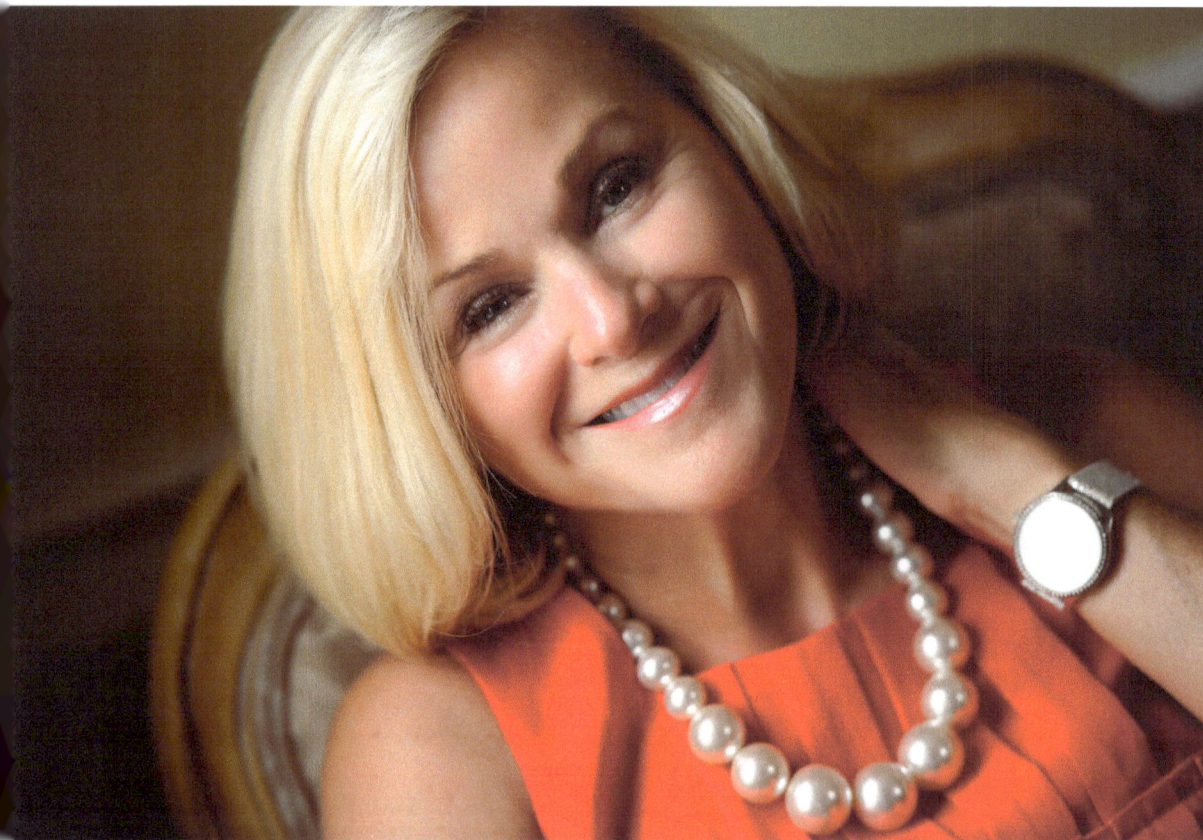

about my grown daughter and the life issues she was facing at this time. Plus, I was working full-time as the Executive Director of the Industrial Authority and Chamber of Commerce, a very demanding position.

When I received this call, no alarms went off – quite the opposite. I've had bad mammograms since I was fairly young, as well as needle aspirations, and these follow-ups were never anything of concern. I actually found my first lump at the age of sixteen. So, I wasn't worried about me. I was worried about everyone around me.

I went in for my second mammogram on January 4th, 2012. The technician showed me the area of concern. It was just a lot of white on the screen, so I was still NOT truly concerned, but followed the instructions to see my regular physician and select a surgeon for a biopsy. The radiologist felt very strongly that I had a lot of DCIS (Ductal Carcinoma In Situ) but not full-blown cancer. After the biopsy and partial

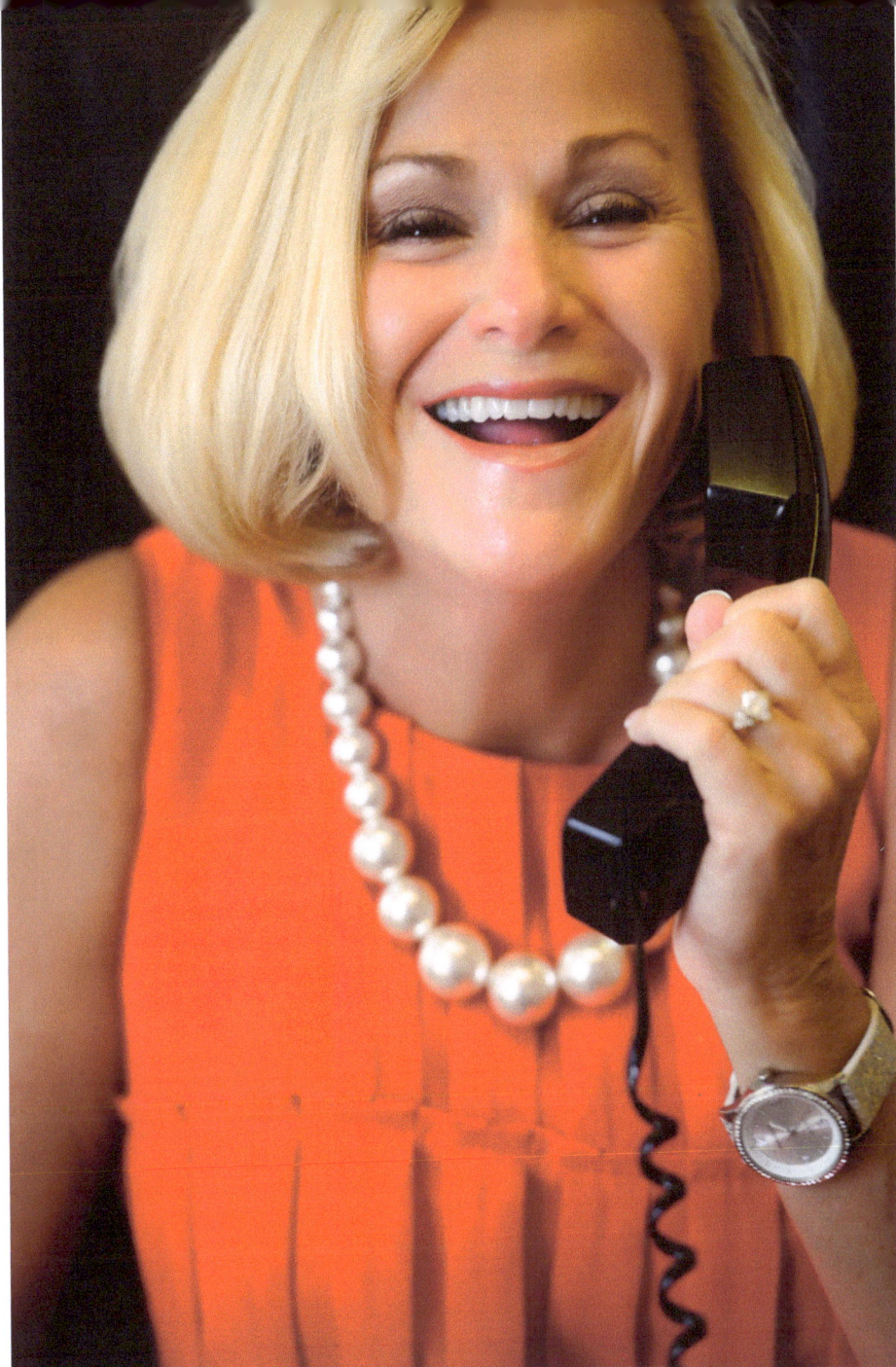

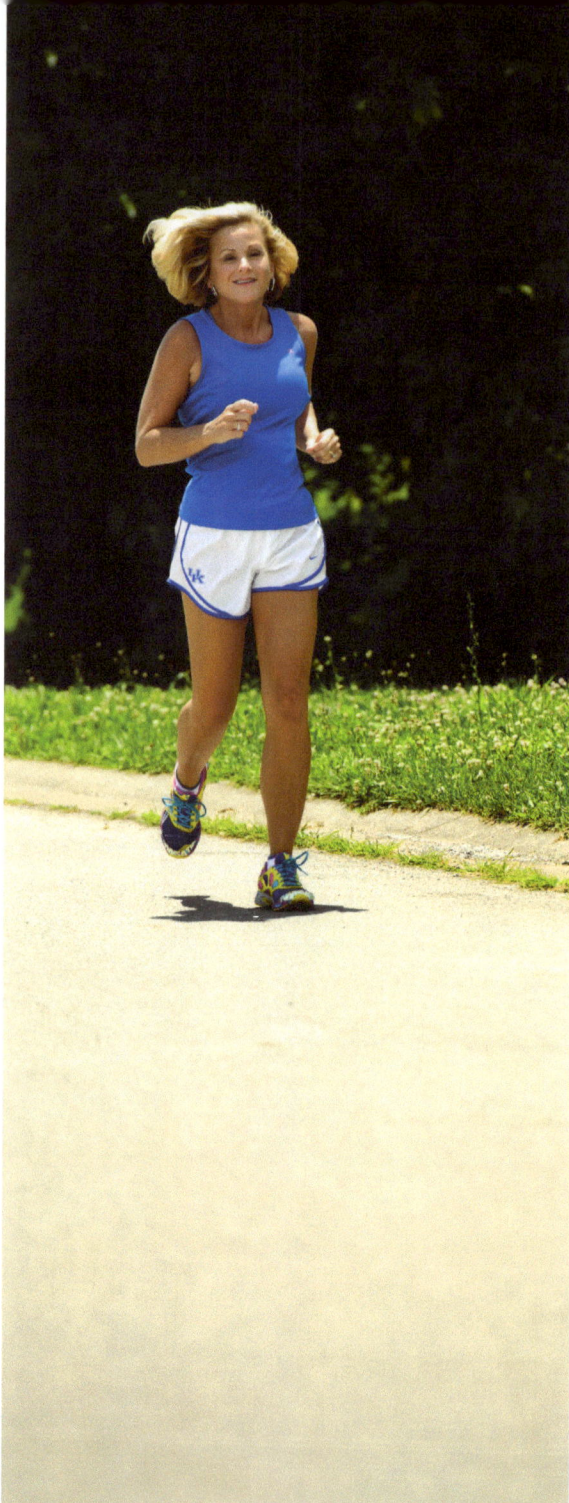

"Cancer made me stop taking my health for granted."

lumpectomy, the results came back.

I was diagnosed with full-blown cancer on February 2nd, 2012.

The surgeon and radiologists both recommended a mastectomy due to the large amount of DCIS. The cancer was small and my surgeon gave me some very good advice: Speak with other women who had been through this and seek their counsel. Every woman I spoke with removed both breasts or said they wished they'd removed both breasts.

With that in mind, I decided to seek out another surgeon, as my first surgeon did not have a plastic surgeon on staff. Feeling that I wanted to remain the woman that I am, I knew I had to have reconstruction. I found a new best friend that had gone through all this (Genea). She recommended her doctors and I moved forward.

I was sitting in my office just a few days before I was scheduled for my bi-lateral mastectomy and was humming a tune in my head. The only words that came to me were, "Cast your cares upon Jesus, look full in his wonderful face".

I remembered hearing my pastor preach a lot about LISTENING to God and he will speak to you through his word or with thoughts in your mind. I had been praying for God to take care of me. I still had a child to raise and a very sick father to help, but as anyone who knows me will tell you, I am talker and a doer but not as good at listening as I should be.

Mid-morning, I decided to go home, pray and listen to God. I needed his reassurance that I was going to be okay. At home, I got on my knees and told God I was ready to listen and asked Him for

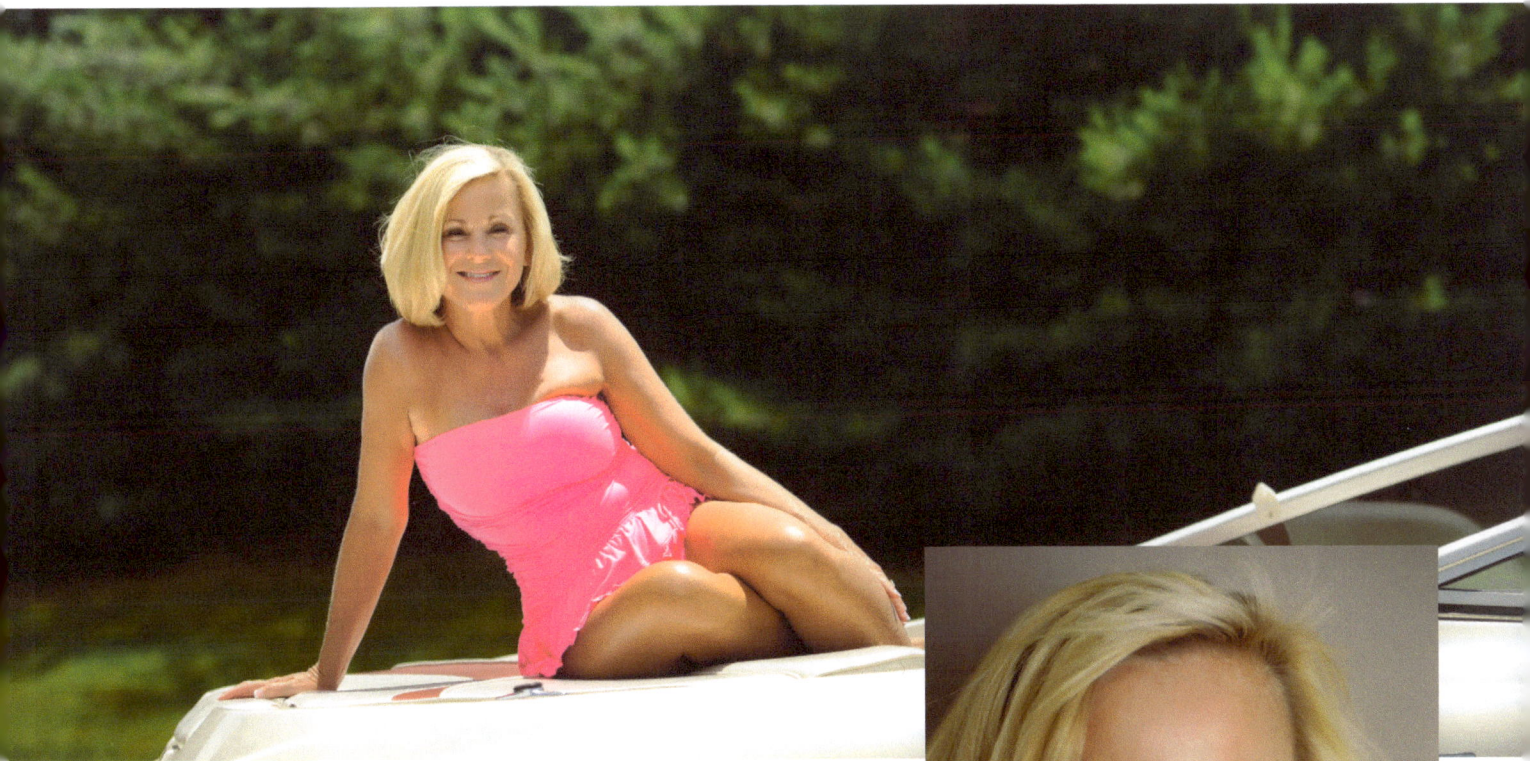

that reassurance I needed.

When I sat in my recliner and opened my bible, it opened to Psalm 55:22: "Cast your cares upon the Lord and he will sustain you; he will never let the righteous be shaken". I knew unequivocally in that moment that my cancer had not spread. It would not be found in my lymph nodes and I was right.

I needed no chemo and I am back to feeling better than ever.

Cancer made me stop taking my health for granted. It taught me to eat better and that what you put into your body is very important. I try to be as healthy as I can!

In today's busy and fast-paced world, it's a challenge to make better choices but I do the very best I can. I run and eat more natural foods like fruits and vegetable and less processed foods. My cancer also made me realize how many caring people there are in this world. Now, I do my best to show others the same care and

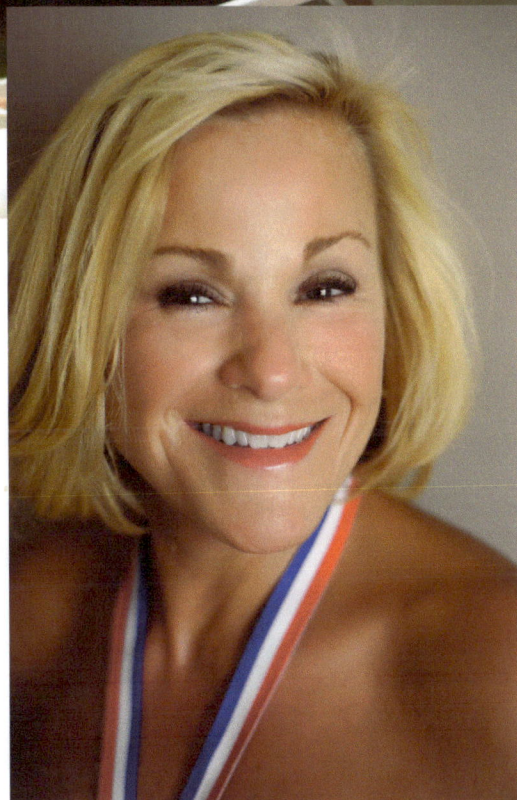

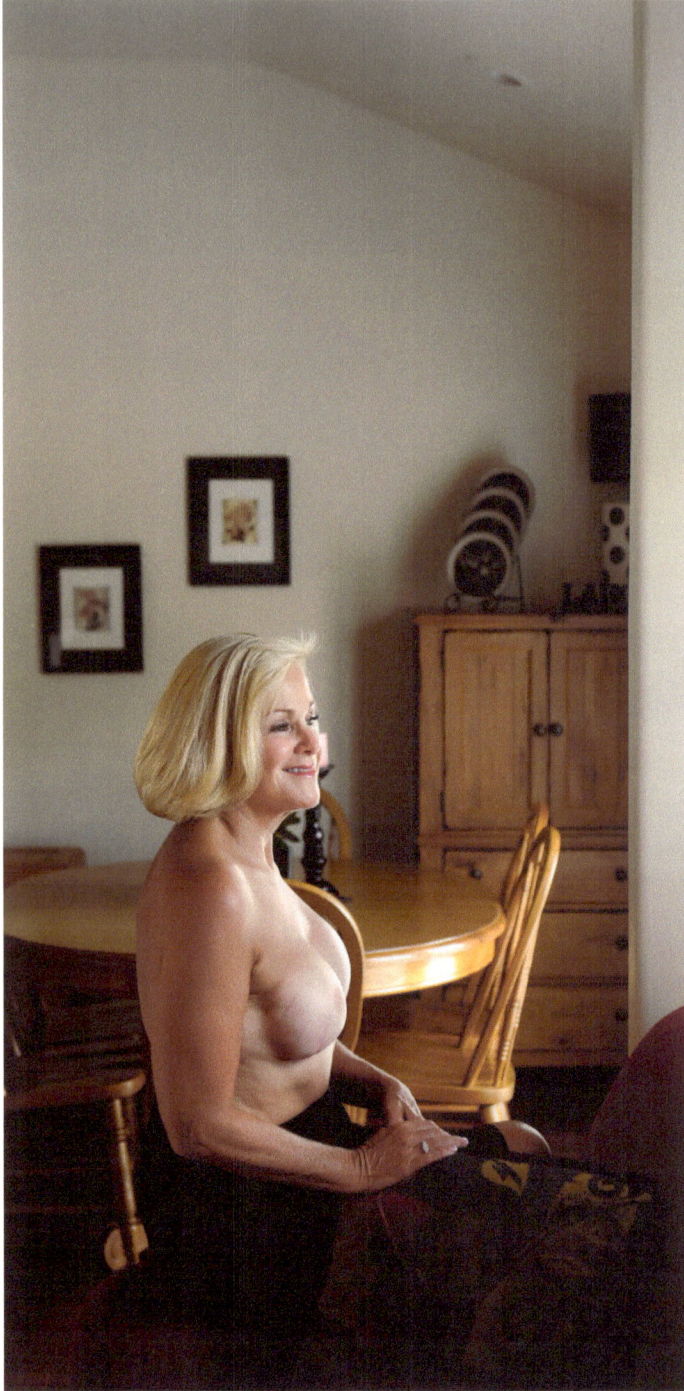
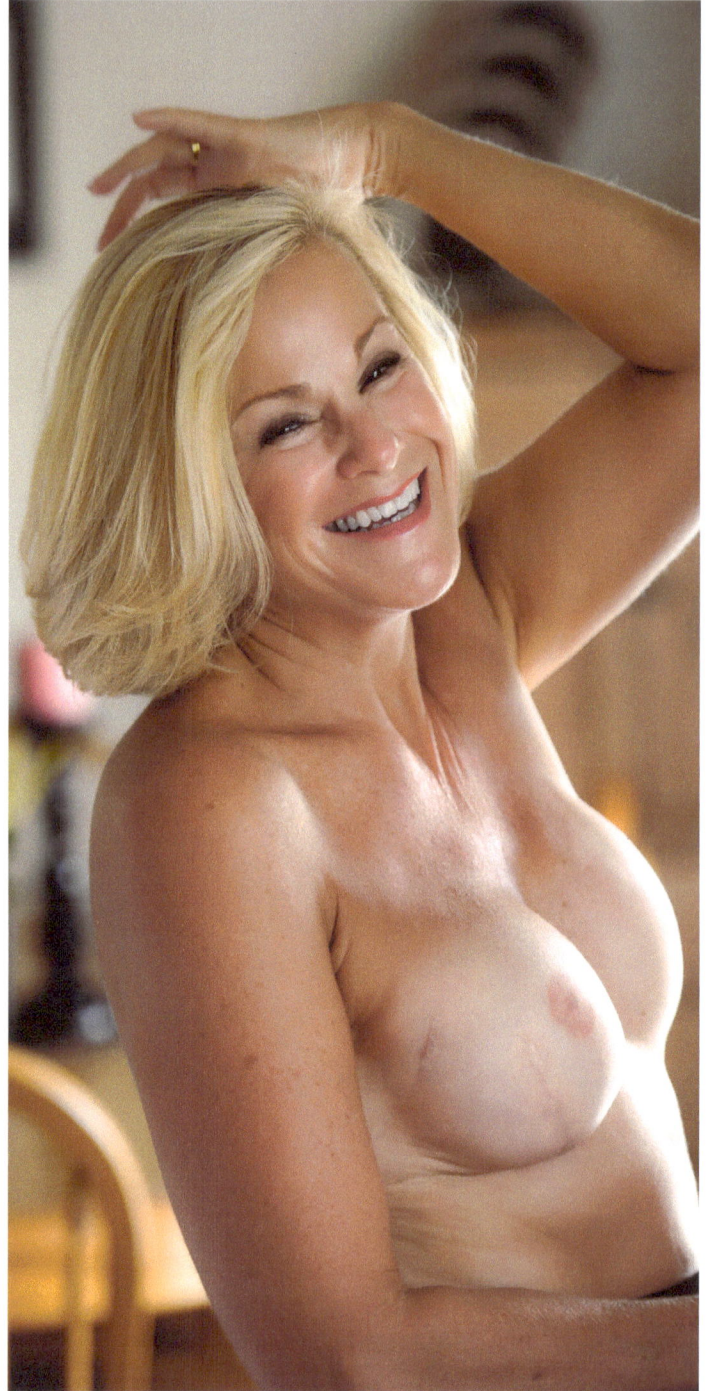

concern that was shown to me.

Through all of this, being a Christian helped me more than anything. "I can do all things through Christ who gives me strength", Philippians 4:13.

God knows what he is doing. I fully relied on Him and He pulled me through.

Life now is better than it was before cancer. I lost my father but know he is in a better place, my grandson's parents are doing much better and helping with him and most of my daughter's issues are being resolved. God had to get me down to teach me to listen to Him and to stop trying to control everything myself.

Cancer was a hurdle on the track of life. Quite frankly, it was not the highest hurdle I have to leap, but leap I did and so can YOU!!!

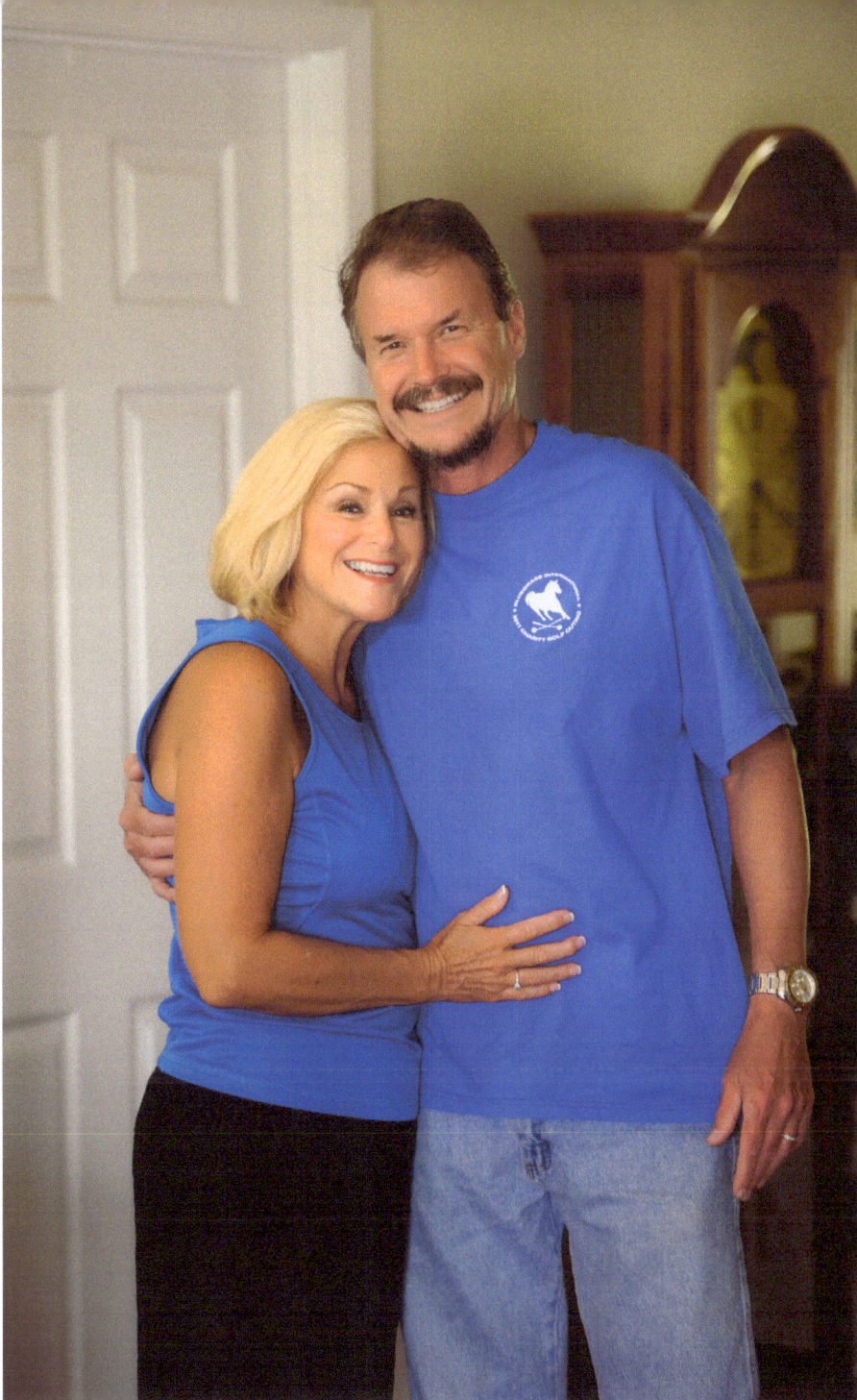

Sherry

March 11th 2009 seemed like just an ordinary evening. My husband and I were lounging around after supper, me on the computer and him in the living room watching TV. The typical evening became anything but when I discovered a lump in my right breast the size of a nickel.

The next morning, I called my gynecologist to set up an appointment. She sent me to see a general surgeon, where the lump was removed. It tested negative for

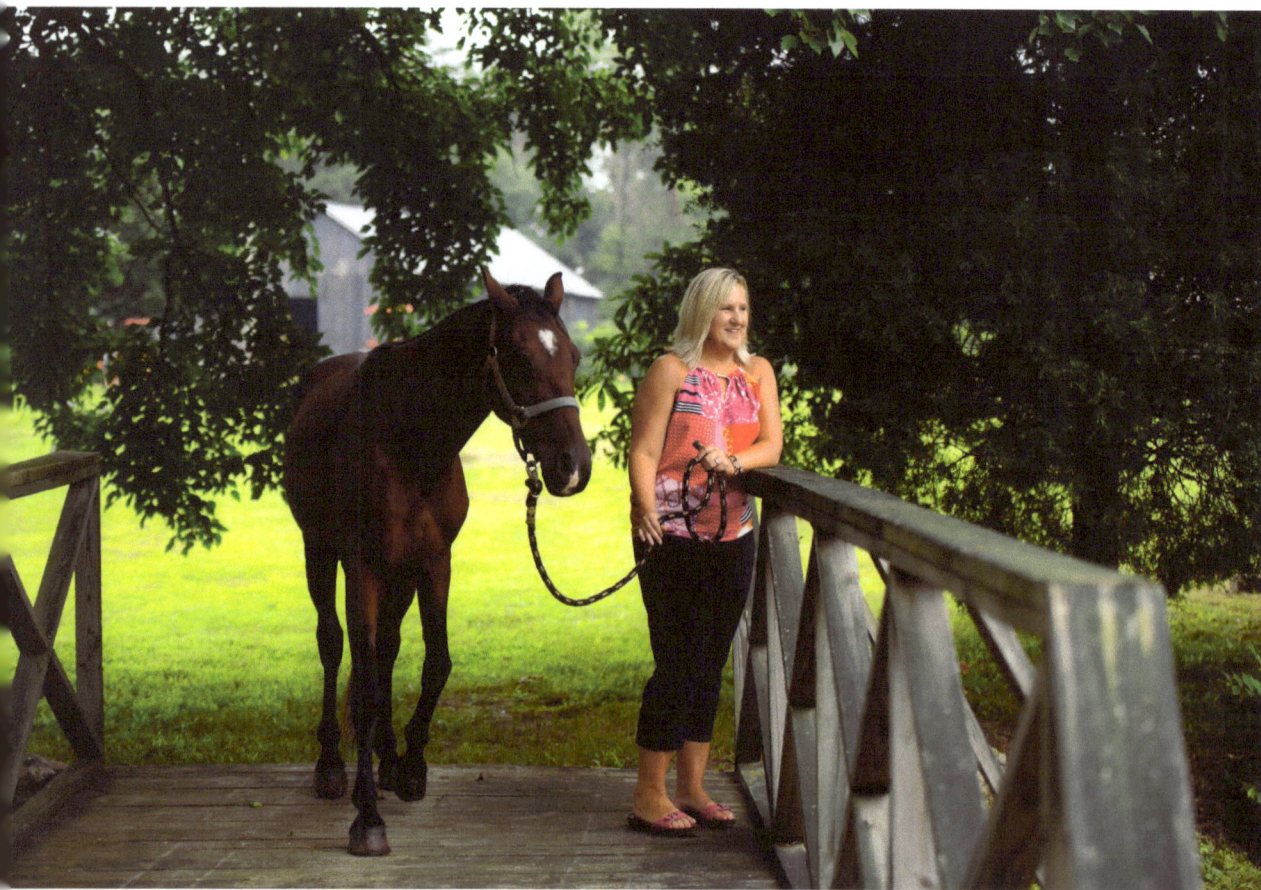

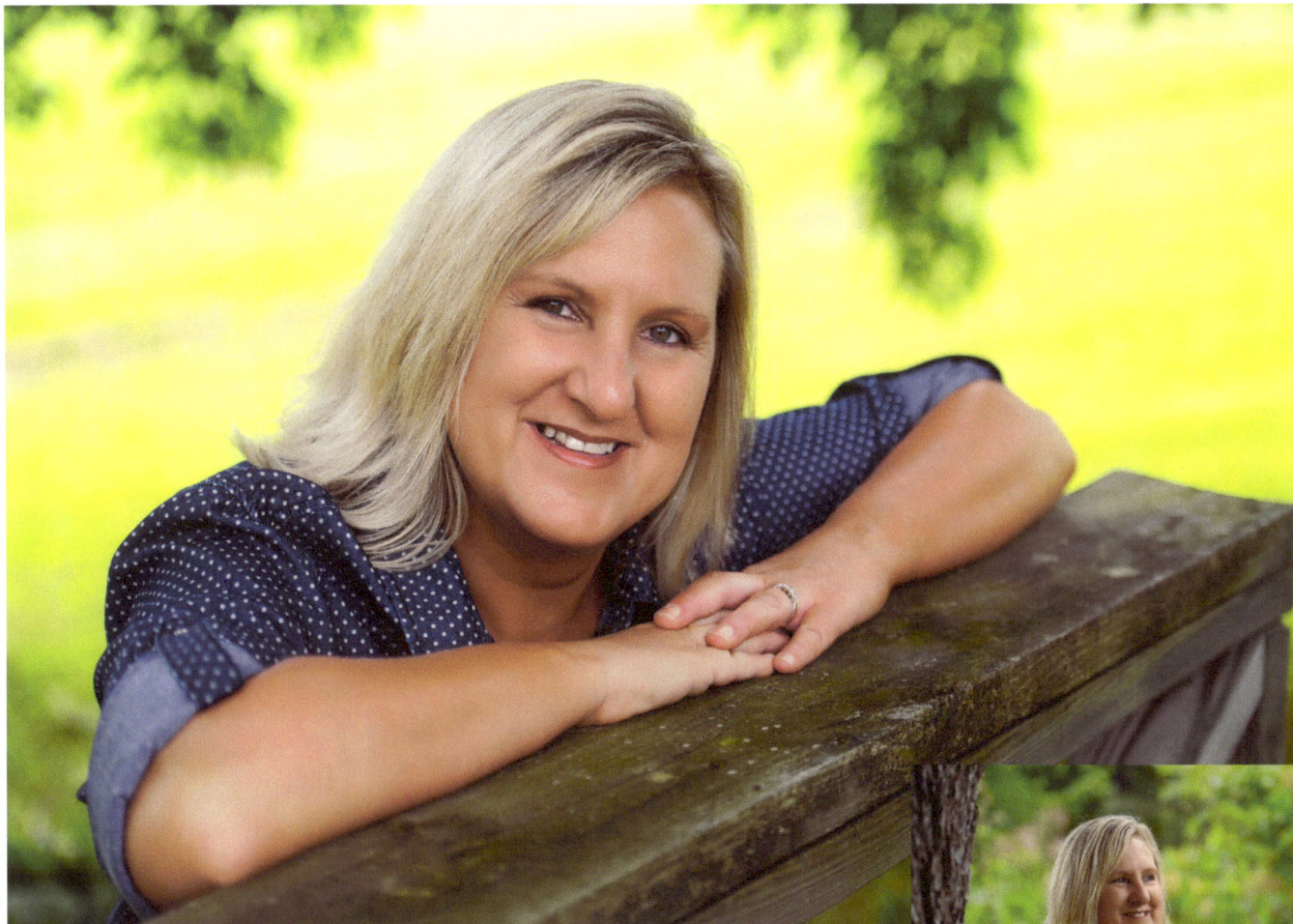

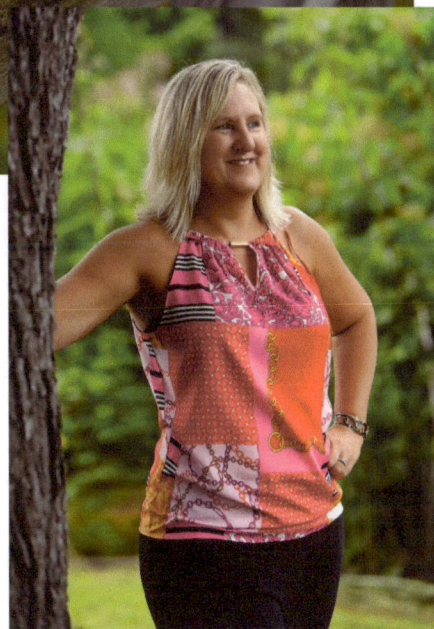

cancer but led to an analysis of other lumps that tested positive.

My husband and I were shocked. We left the office in tears. I was only thirty-six! It didn't make sense that cancer was now looming over our heads. Just a few days before, we'd purchased the home of our dreams.

Joe made the phone calls to our family, starting with my mother. Our family was so supportive. In spite of how helpless we felt, they were certain I could beat this disease.

The next few weeks were a blur of tests and decisions.

Tests revealed precancerous cells on both breasts. The hospital recommended a surgeon to perform a double mastectomy and a plastic surgeon to perform reconstruction. From there, I

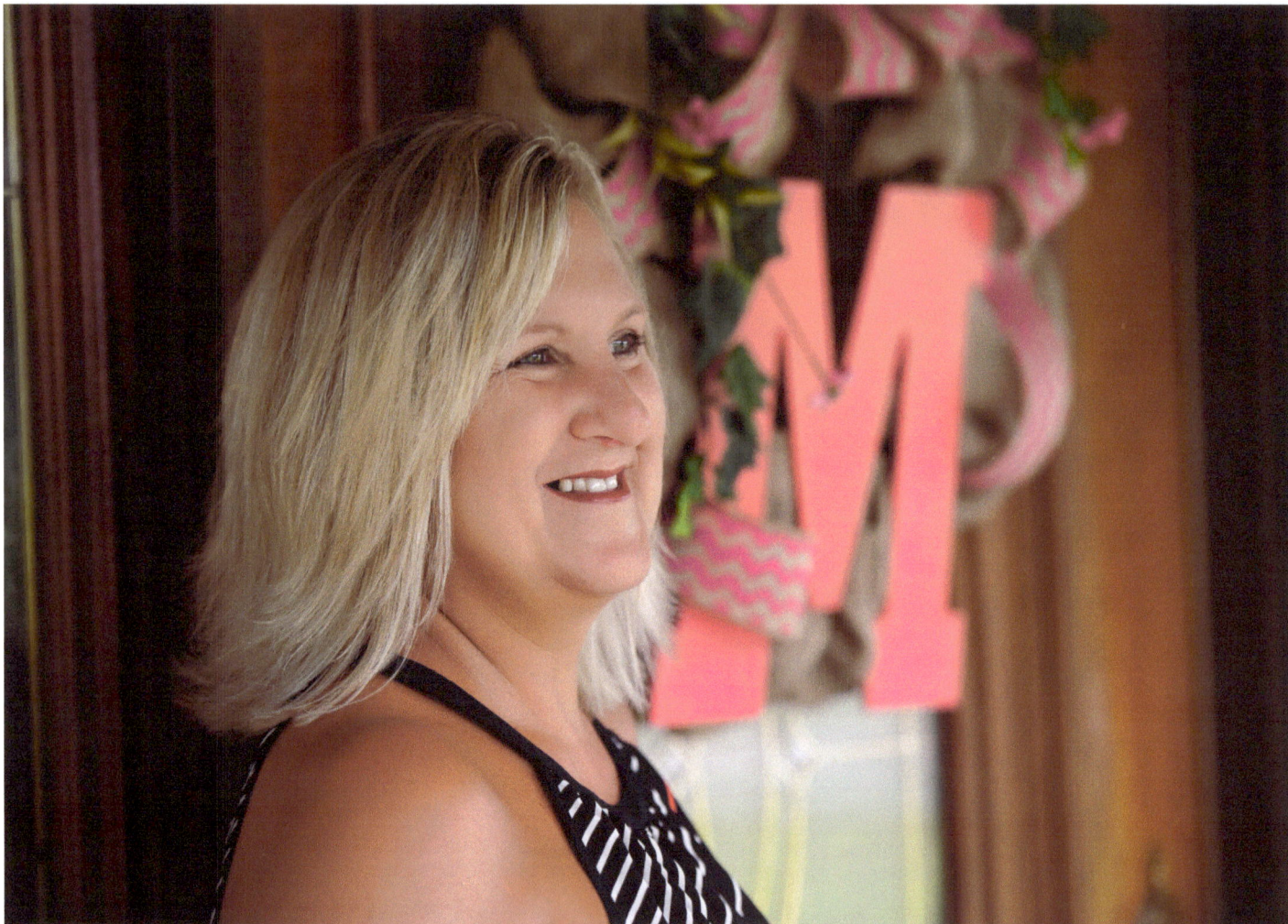

would have to find an oncologist to treat the cancer.

This seemed so backwards. Wouldn't it make sense to treat the cancer first then worry about the rest? Joe and I decided to visit the oncologist, where I asked him about removing my breast.

The oncologist said something that we still consider the only funny thing to come out of this experience: "If you see me with a scalpel then you had better run." He then explained that the double mastectomy and reconstruction surgery should come first, followed by test results and numbers to determine how to best treat the cancer.

We set an appointment for the double mastectomy, followed by a meeting with the plastic surgeon. There, I learned that my plastic surgeon would be present during the surgery, mark where she wanted the surgeon to make incisions and, once the breasts were removed, place tissue expanders to help keep the space. I was much more comfortable with the idea of the surgery once I knew the exact process. I was not going to lose my breasts knowing they could be reconstructed at the same time as the mastectomies!

The surgery for the double mastectomy and immediate reconstruction went well. It only lasted a few hours and my family was there to support me. The next day, I returned home to our brand new house where my family and friends were waiting. They welcomed me with words of encouragement and the healing process began.

Post-operatively, I began to visit my plastic surgeon to continue the process of reconstructing my breasts. My self-esteem and confidence were low following the double mastectomy and her staff was truly the best. They helped me feel like I'd made the right

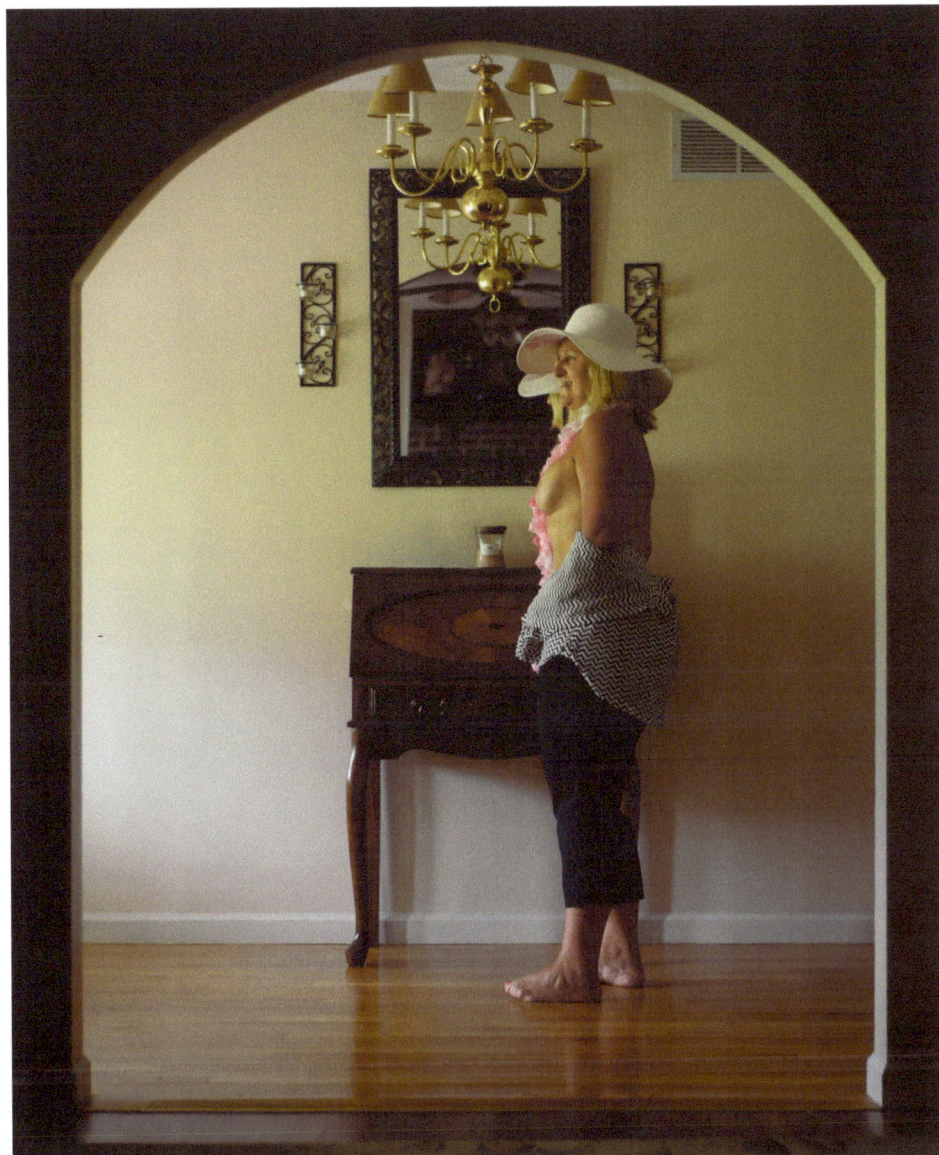

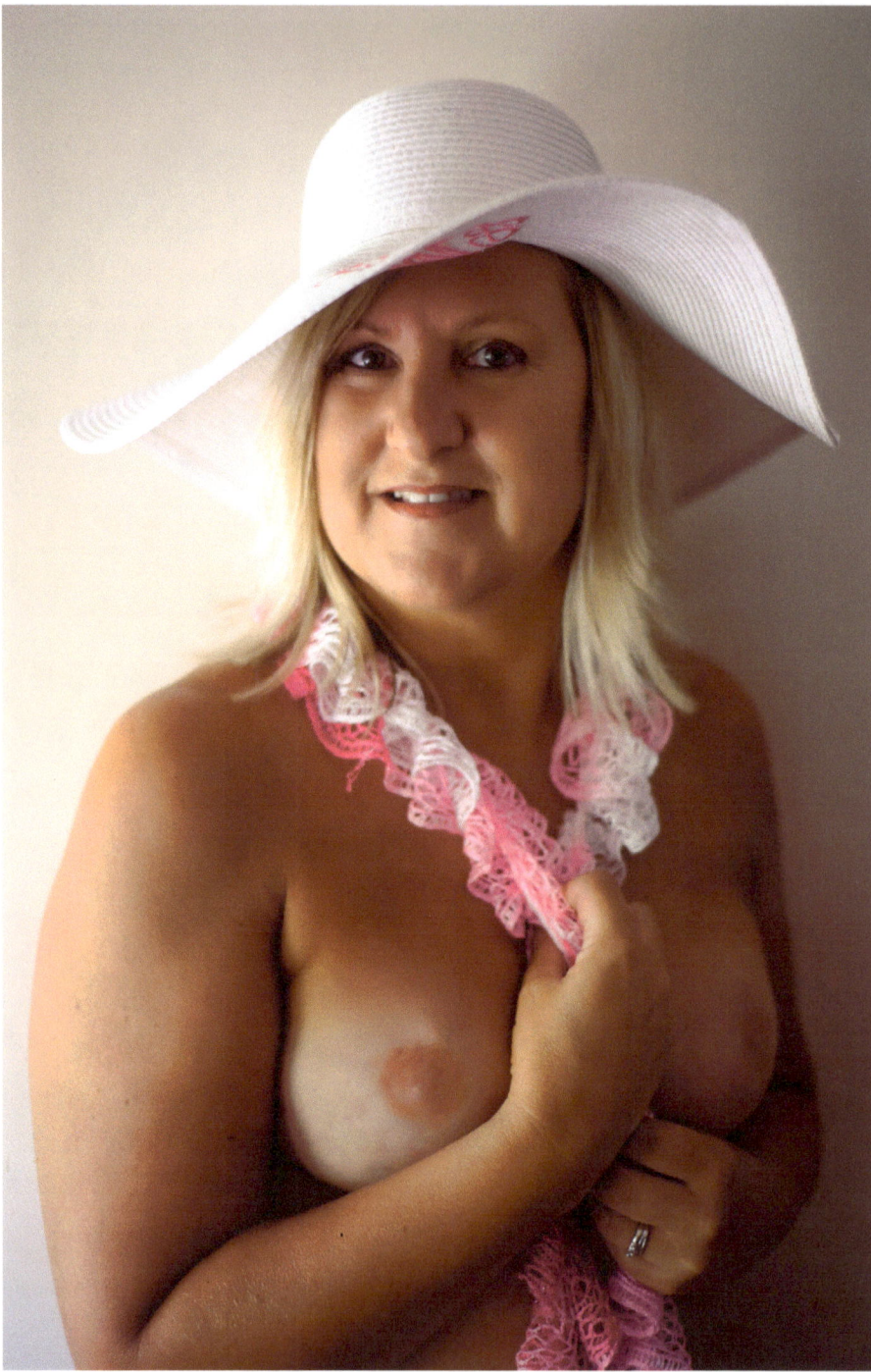

"Never, ever give up."

decision. After each weekly visit, as my breasts started to take shape, I felt happier and more positive.

I also received good news during my first visit to the oncologist: the number (or the size) of cancer that I had in my lumps and lymph nodes would not require chemo or radiation. My husband and I were so grateful for that news. I was placed on Tamoxifin.

Unfortunately, this wasn't the end of my journey. The oncologist recommended a PET scan to ensure the cancer had not spread. A cancerous spot was spotted on one of my ovaries. Treatment then required the removal of my ovaries and a change in my cancer medication.

In the meantime, the reconstruction of my breasts turned out great! My plastic surgeon was able to save my right nipple and grafted it below my belly button. A little weird at first to see my nipple was below my belly button, but I knew this was only temporary and it would be relocated to where it should be at the appropriate time. The nipple was eventually split in half and transferred to where they belonged over each

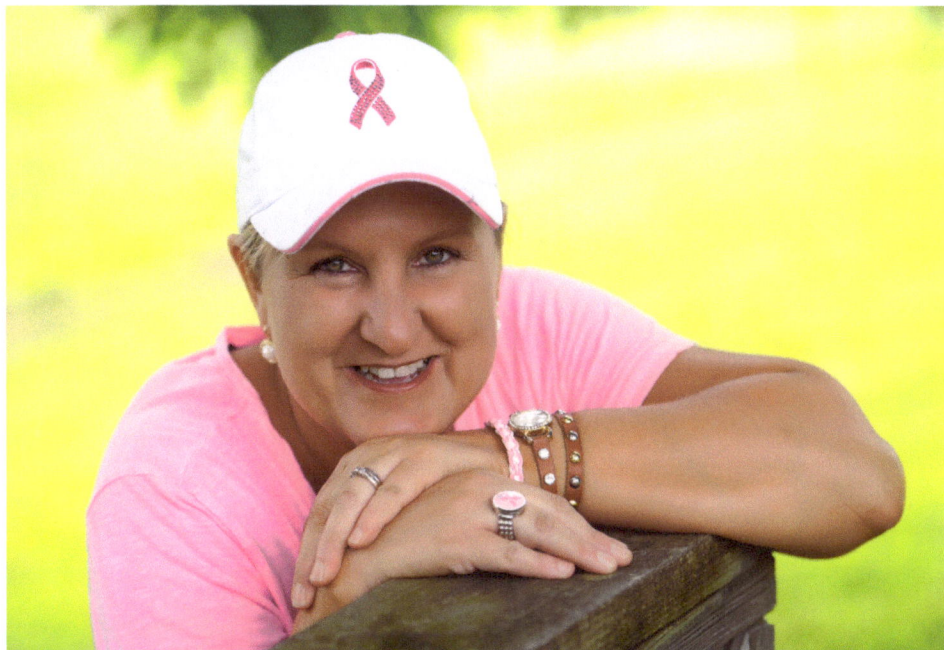

of my breasts. The nipples even retained their ability to react to pressure and temperature!! (Who would have ever thought that would have worked?) Areolas were also tattooed on each of my breasts to give them a more natural look.

On May 30, 2013, my husband and I returned for a check-up with the general surgeon who had performed the double mastectomy. It went great! The doctor actually released me from ever coming back to see him, which made Joe and I so happy.

In June 2014, I will be five years out from cancer. My husband and I can hardly wait for that date. Not only will it be a huge relief, the five-year marker will represent a major accomplishment.

Today, we are active members of Relay for Life. We have a lot more pink   in   our lives than we did four years ago. We plan to "Rock the Ribbon and Keep Believing!"

We hope that others struggling with breast cancer will remember this: Never, ever give up. Let everyone around you help. Always keep your head up and believe in the power of prayer.

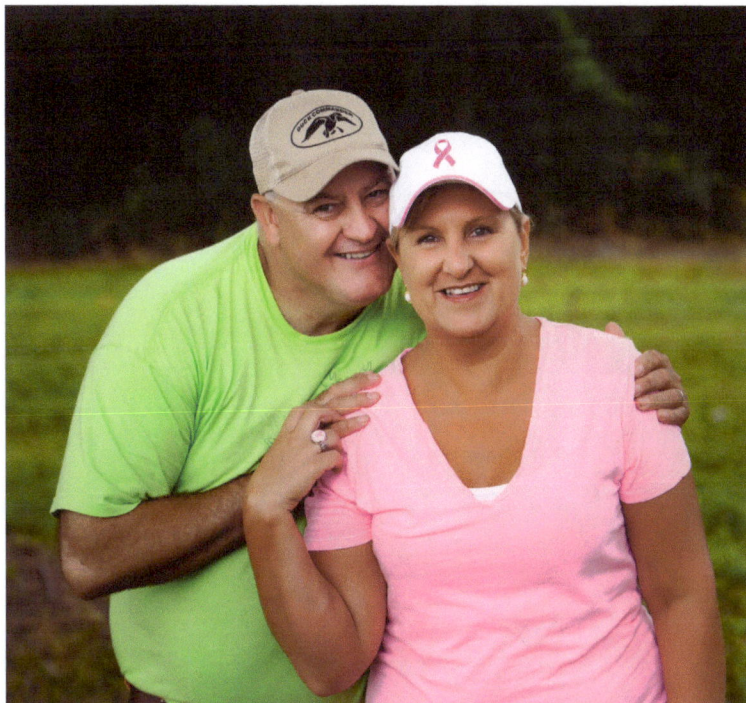

Beverly

My mother was diagnosed with breast cancer when I was twenty-eight years old. The doctor treating her suggested that my sisters and I should have a baseline mammogram to see if the disease might be affecting more of us.

I waited almost a year to schedule mine. Perhaps it was because I didn't believe I could have breast cancer at the young age of twenty-eight. Or maybe I did not want to hear the diagnosis

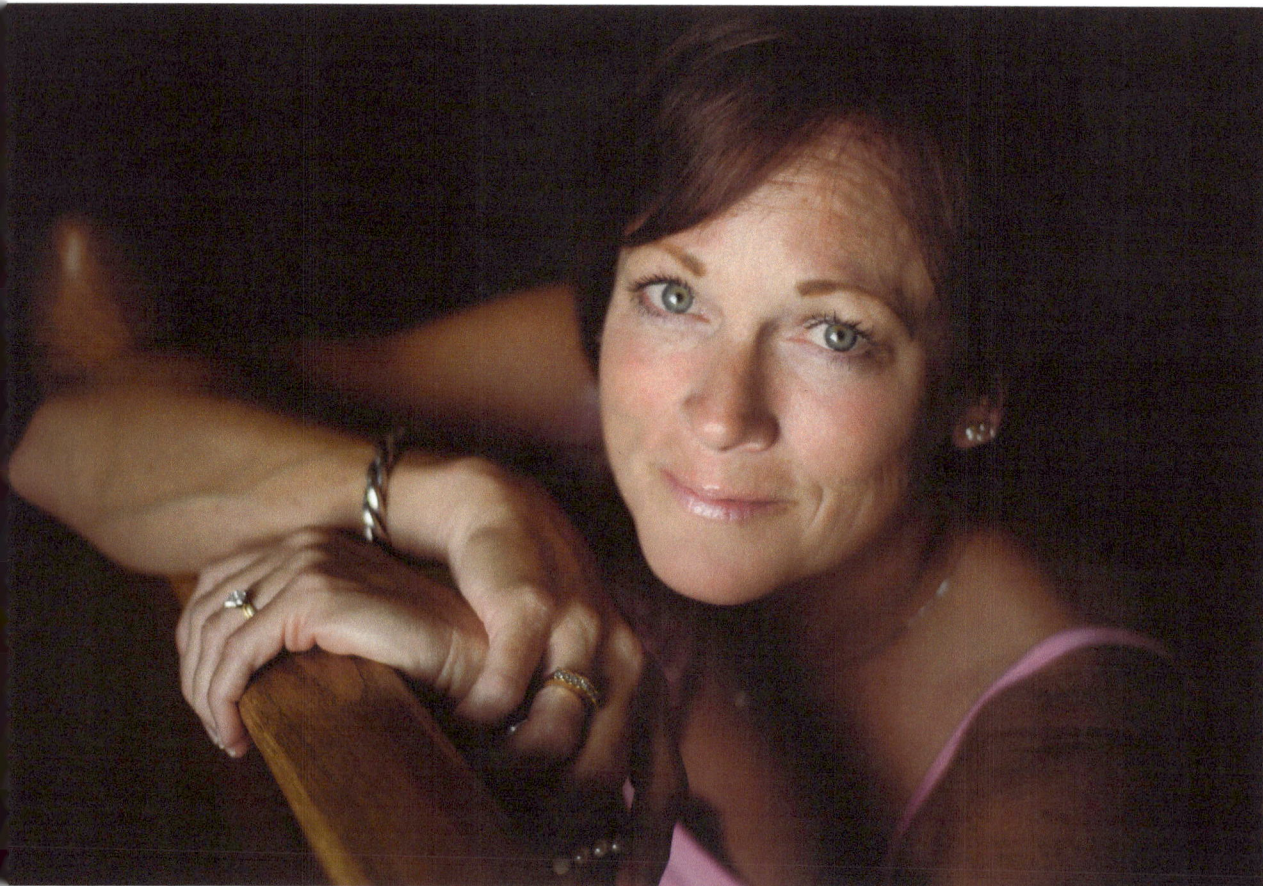

because I was nervous that I did.

In March of 1992, I summoned up the courage to have a mammogram. Once that was done, I headed to work. A routine day - and my life in general - changed when I received a phone call from my doctor: "There is an area on your right breast and I would like for you to see a surgeon for a biopsy".

"Ok, it's probably nothing", I thought, and did my best to put it out of my mind. I met with a surgeon very soon after and scheduled the biopsy.

I remember the ride with my mother to get the results. My thoughts were that she had done this, and if I had to, I could too.

I was called into a room some time later and the doctor walked in and gave me the results: "You have cancer."

Wow! The enormity of that statement sank in pretty quick. Ok, this was real now, no "ifs". "Biopsy", "lumpectomy", "chemo-

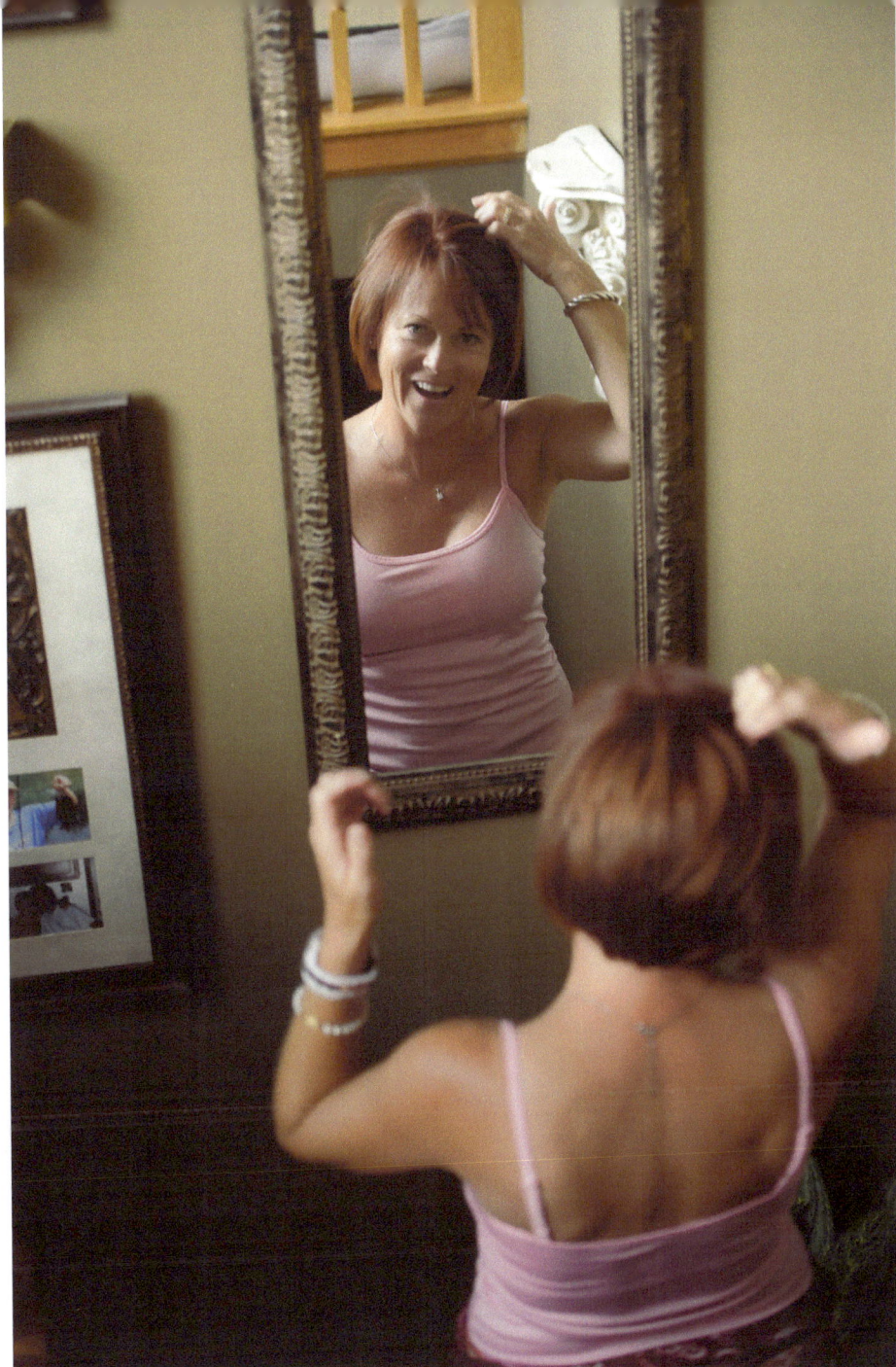

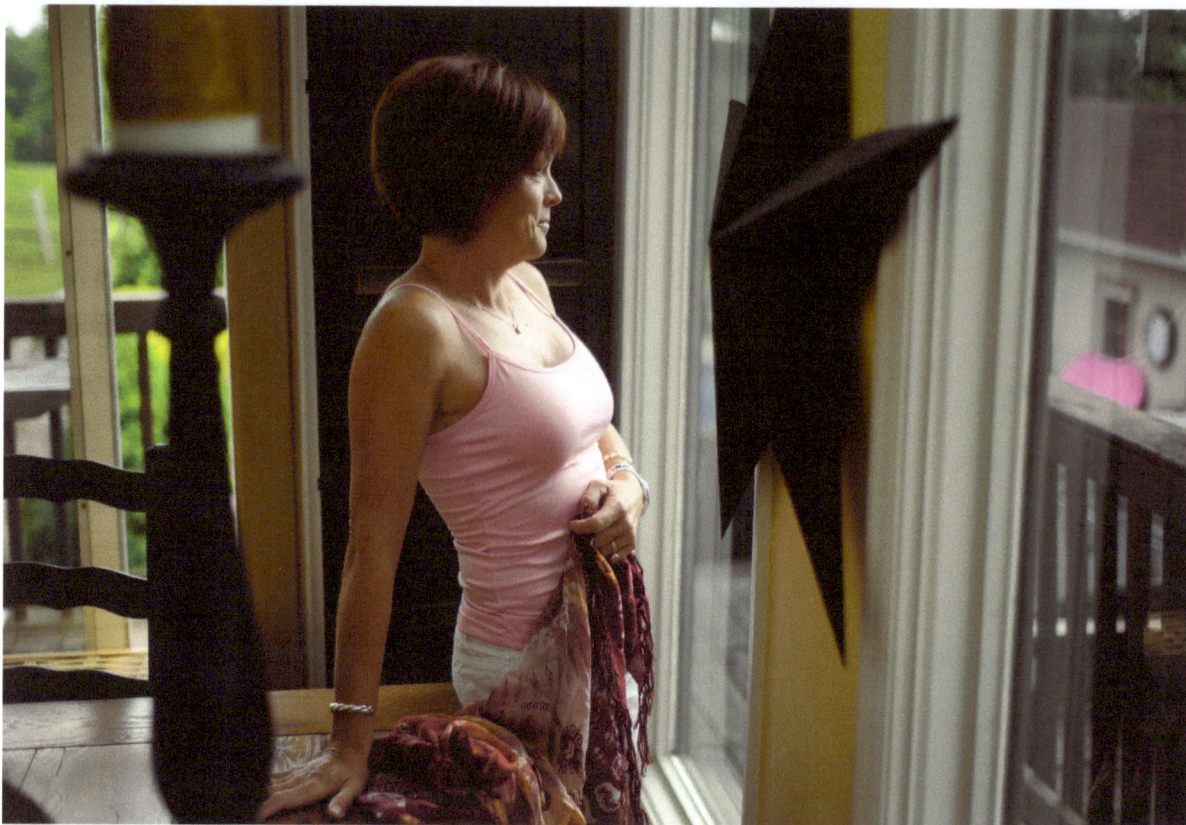

therapy", "radiation" were words no one ever wants to hear - let alone experience - but I did.

At times the treatment was brutal, the anxiety was always great, and the fear was always present. But, with my mother there to guide and support me, along with the rest of my family, I completed my treatments. From there, I headed into a future in which the ugly word "cancer" would always and forever be a part of.

That was 1992.

During this time, my family was not my only support. Soon after my lumpectomy I started dating a guy who actually wanted to go to my treatments with me. My cancer didn't scare him, and he was with me through chemotherapy, radiation and after! Soon after I completed my treatment, he proposed.

We were married in the fall of 1993.

Just over a year after that, on Christmas Eve, I lost my mother to metastatic breast cancer. I think of her often, on her birthday and the date of her death, as well as the dates of her diagnosis as well as my own. In a strange way, her diagnosis

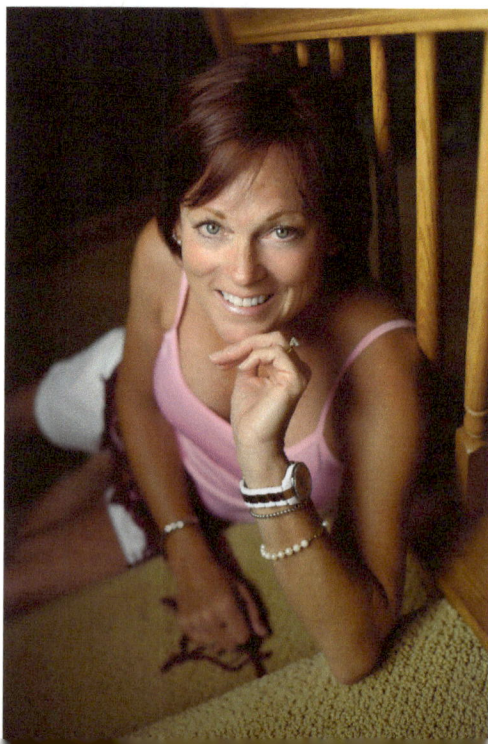

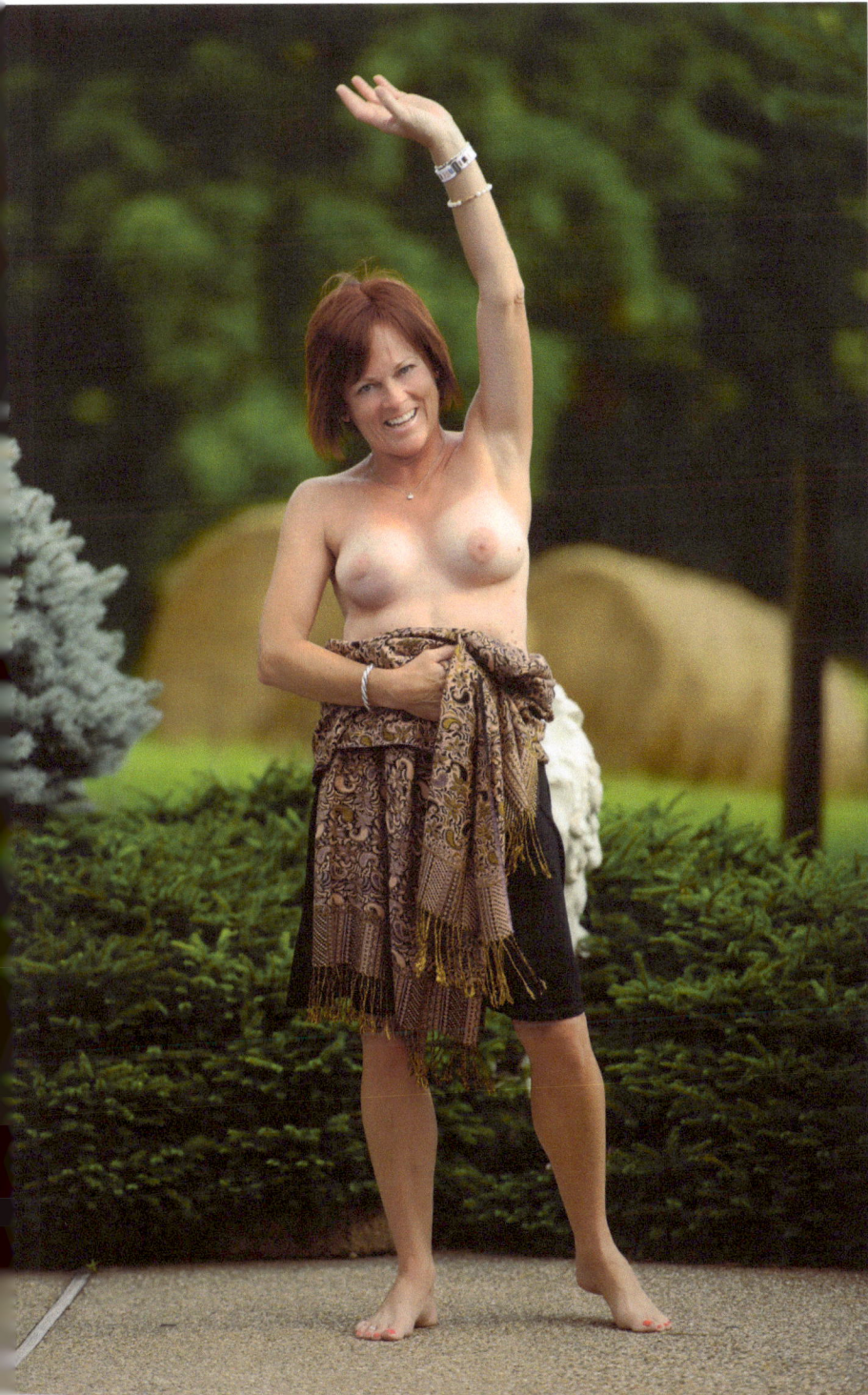

"*I have been happier with the results than I could have expected!*"

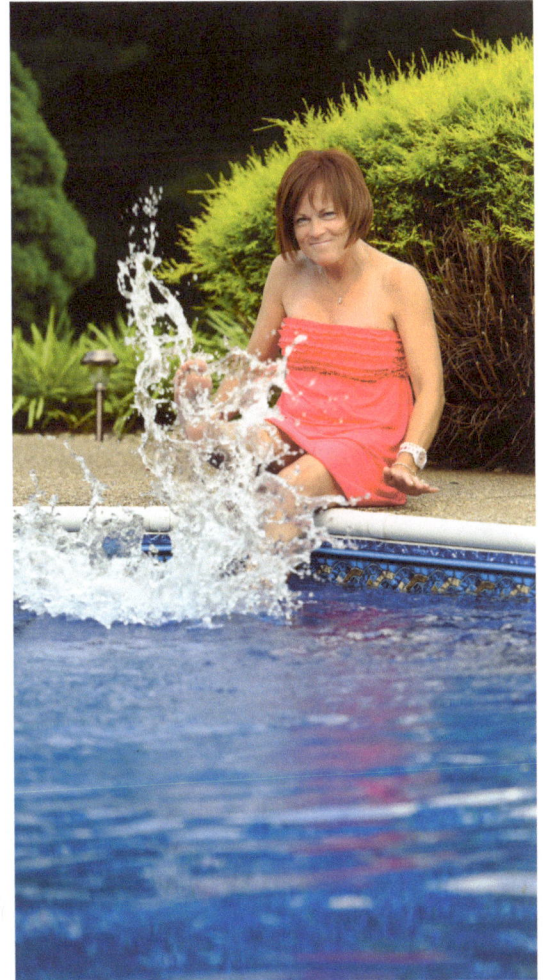

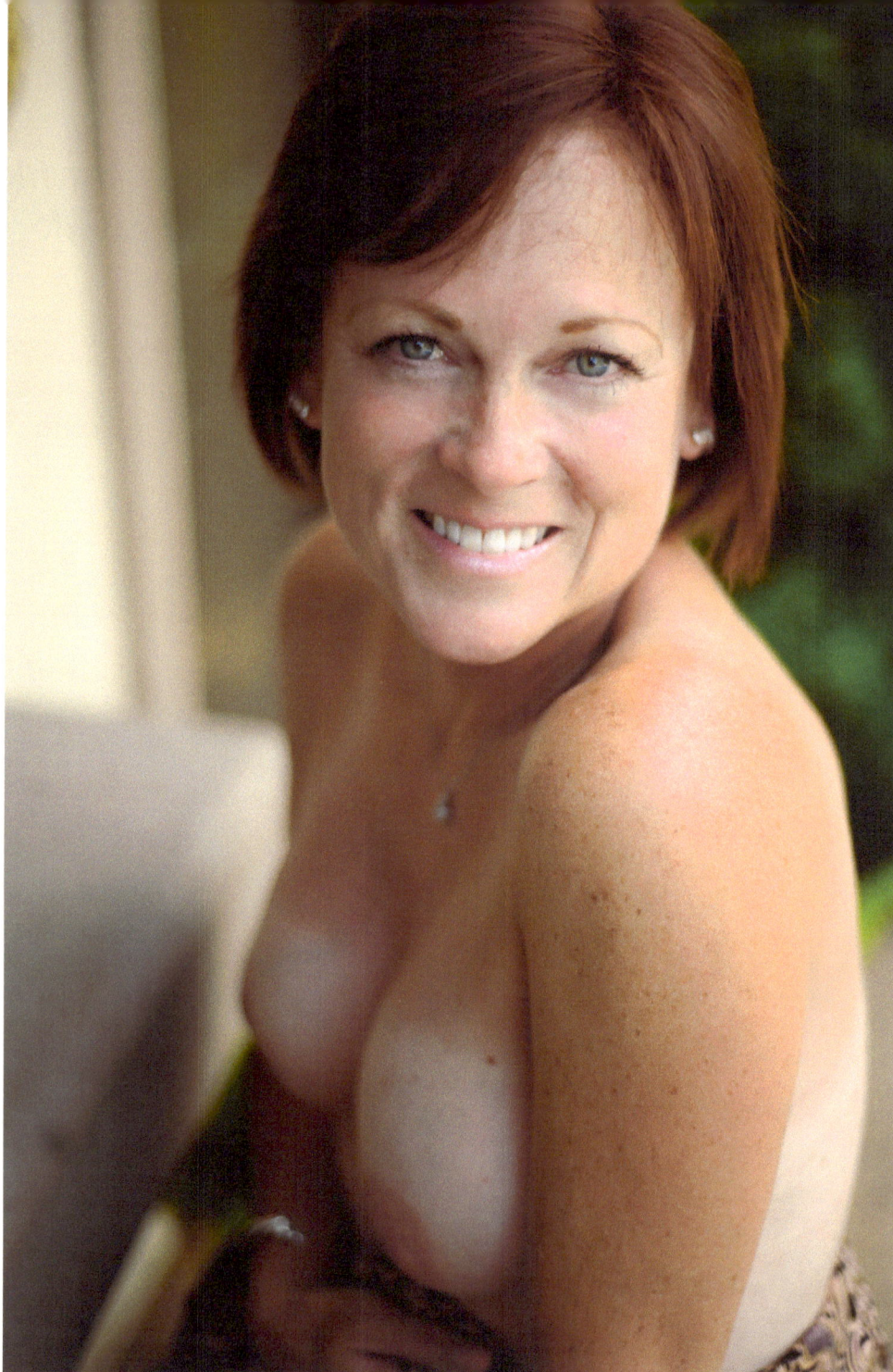

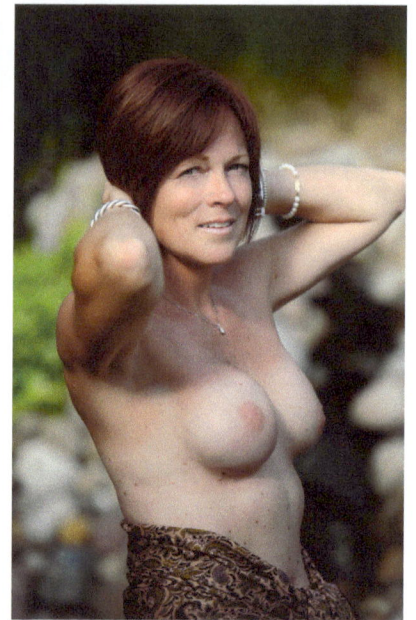

saved my life.

I have been blessed with two children. They know about my battle with cancer. They are being raised to understand the importance of prevention and early detection. My daughter is sixteen and my son is fourteen, and they know they will have to endure their own respective cancer screenings, but they also know that screening and treatment are the reasons their mother is still with them.

Over the last twenty years, I have had two additional biopsies (both benign) on the same side. After my last biopsy, I decided I wanted to have reconstructive surgery to "even" out my chest so I could wear sweaters or not feel self-conscious in tops.

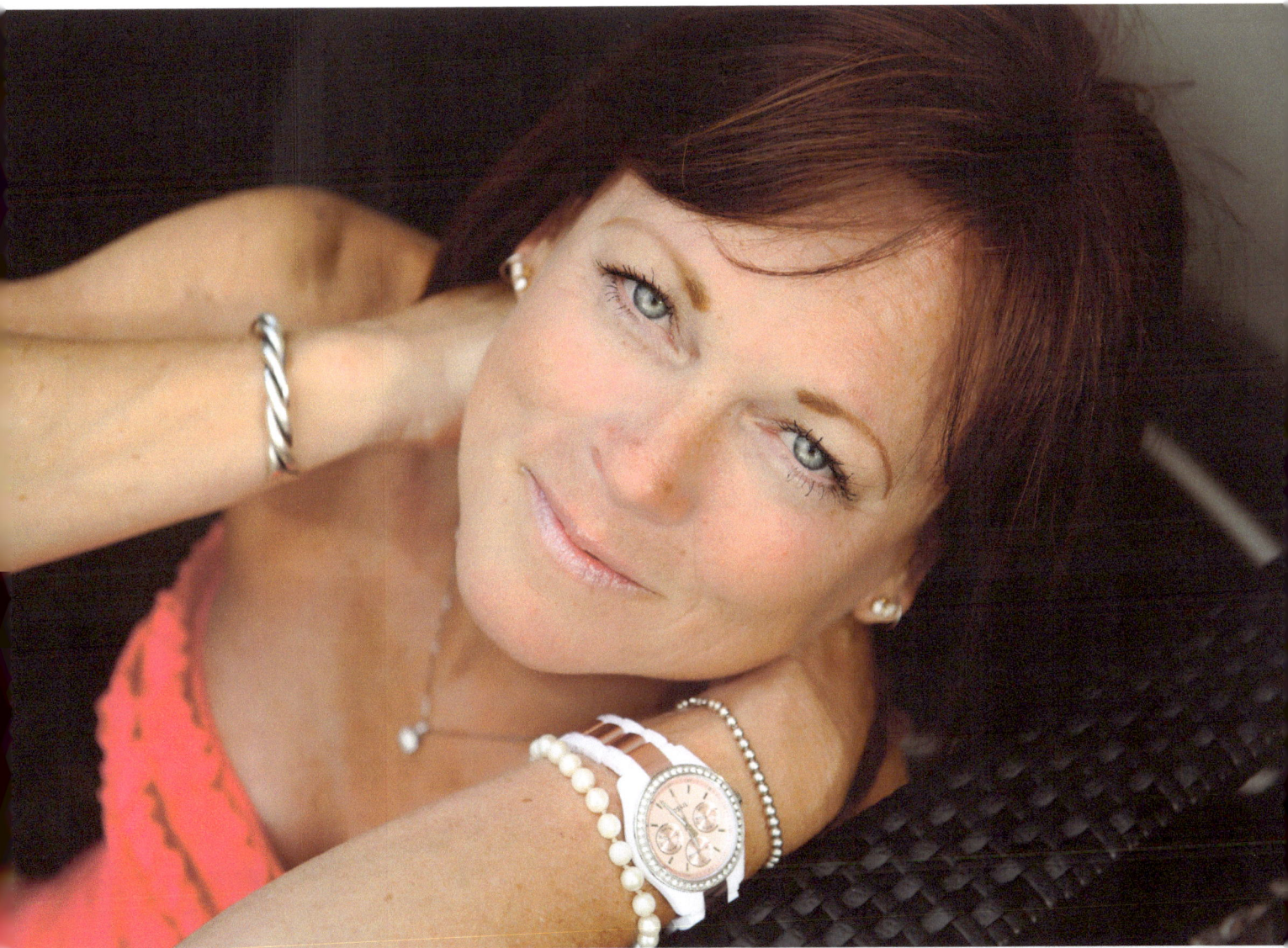

I was referred to a plastic surgeon that was extremely sympathetic to my feelings. She understood how a healthy body image is an important part of overcoming cancer and was a fantastic partner in helping me to undo some of the effects cancer has had on my body.

I have been happier with the results than I could have expected!

Jill

My name is Jill. I was diagnosed with breast cancer in Dec of 2011. Here's my story:

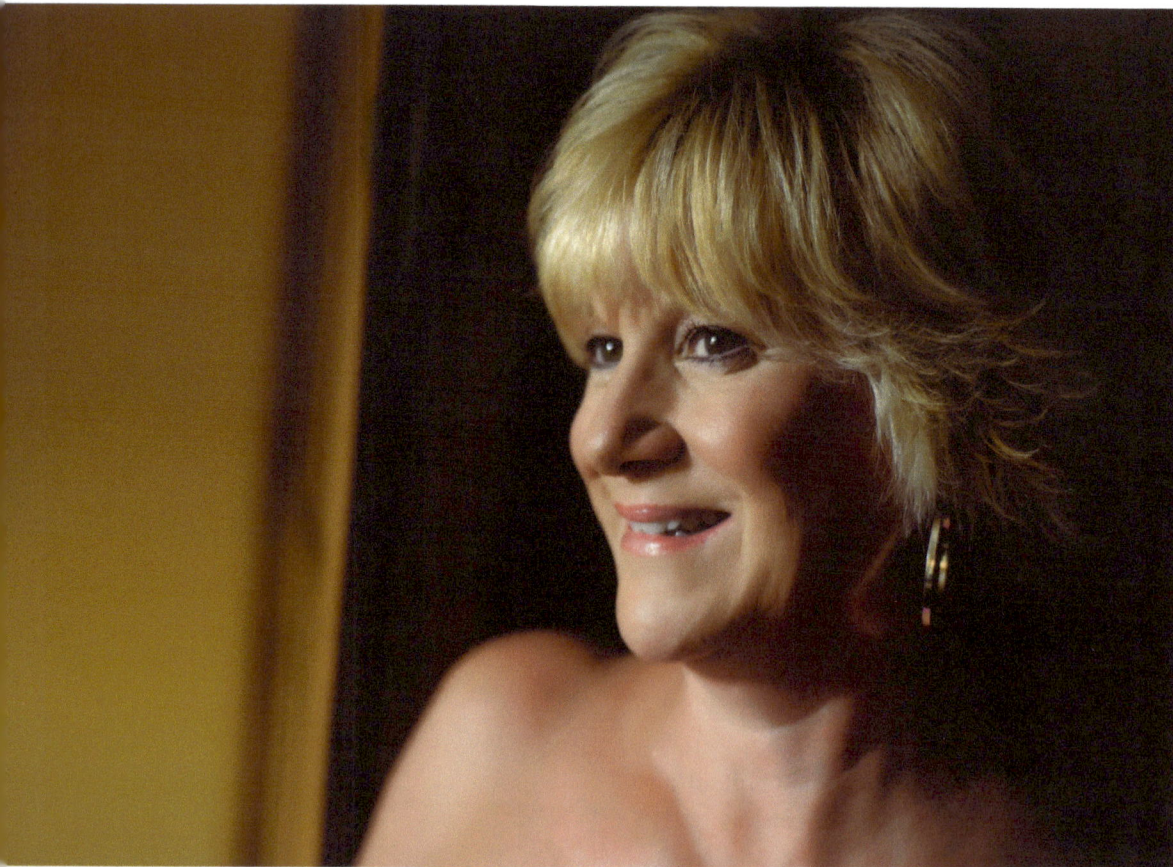

It's not always gloom and doom.

There can be good results after a mastectomy if you have informative people around you like I did. I was also very thankful to have my wonderful and caring husband, David, lots of family members and a special friend, Celia. She was always there for me, cheering me on.

I was very blessed to work with an observant and knowledgeable gynecologist. He didn't agree with the results of a mammogram and ultra sound. It was diagnosed as Nothing, No

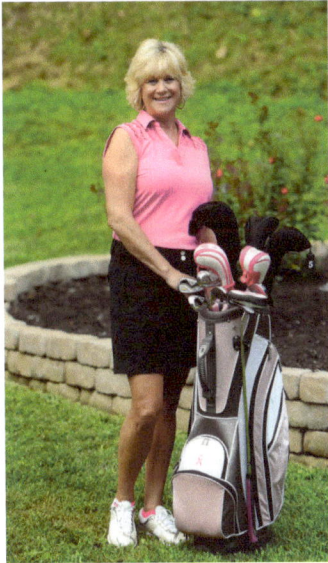

Signs of Breast Cancer, See you in a year!

My gynecologist wanted a second opinion, especially since my niece was diagnosed with breast cancer at the age of thirty and passed away at thirty-two. So, after many biopsies and finally a MRI, I was diagnosed with breast cancer.

The journey began.

I went to a surgeon and he assured me that all I needed was a lumpectomy. This process would require the removal of my entire nipple. Thank goodness I learned about my options, including the option to see a plastic surgeon.

I asked my surgeon's office for some names of plastic surgeons they would recom-

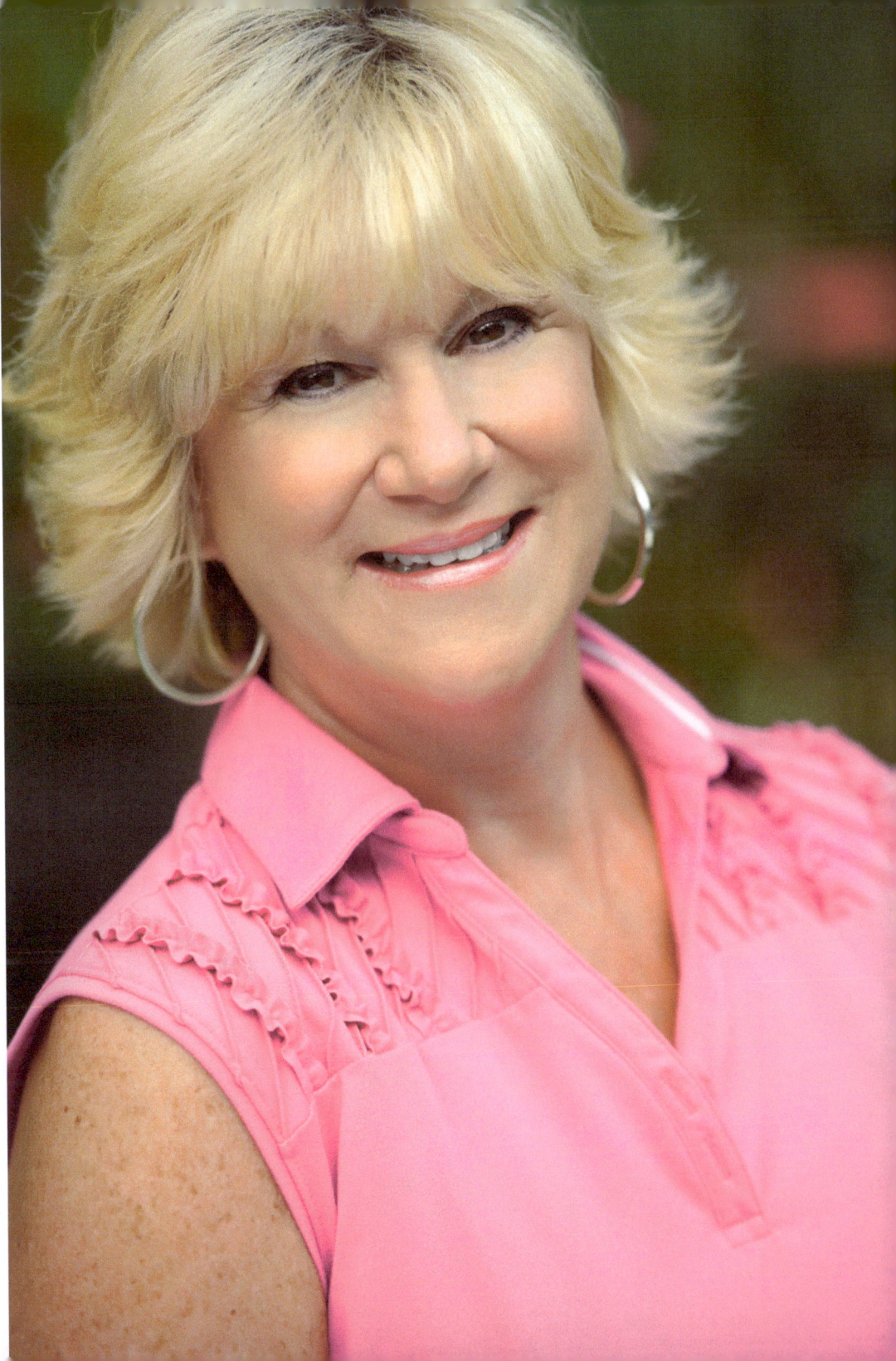

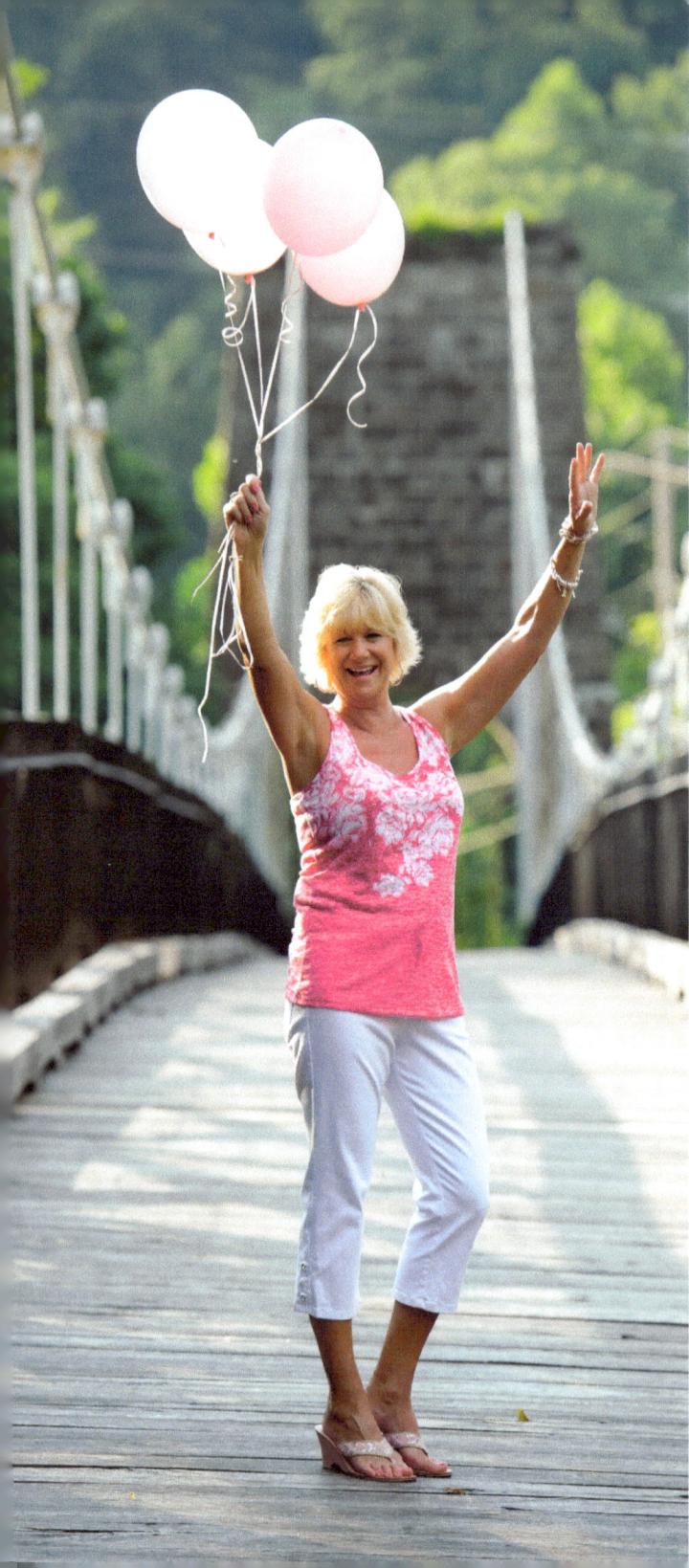

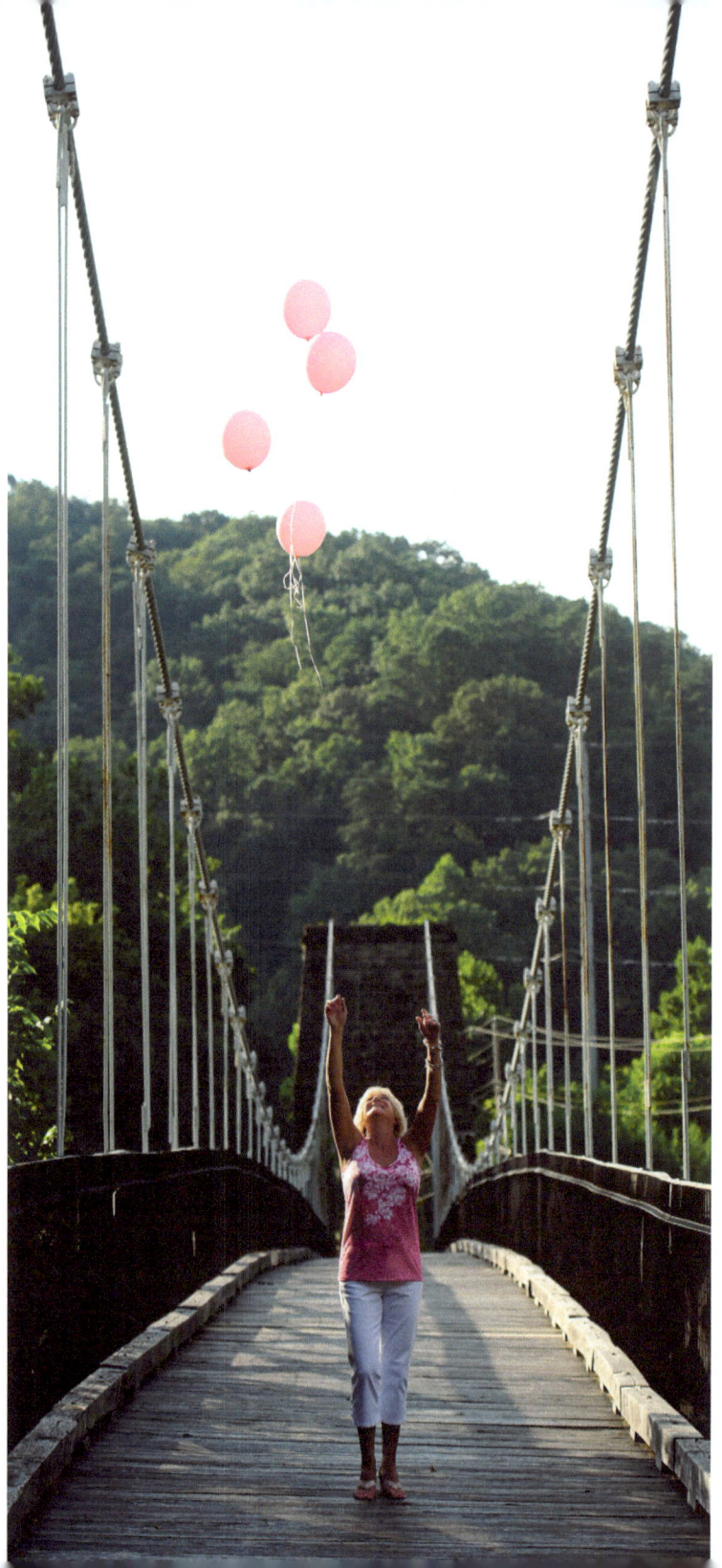

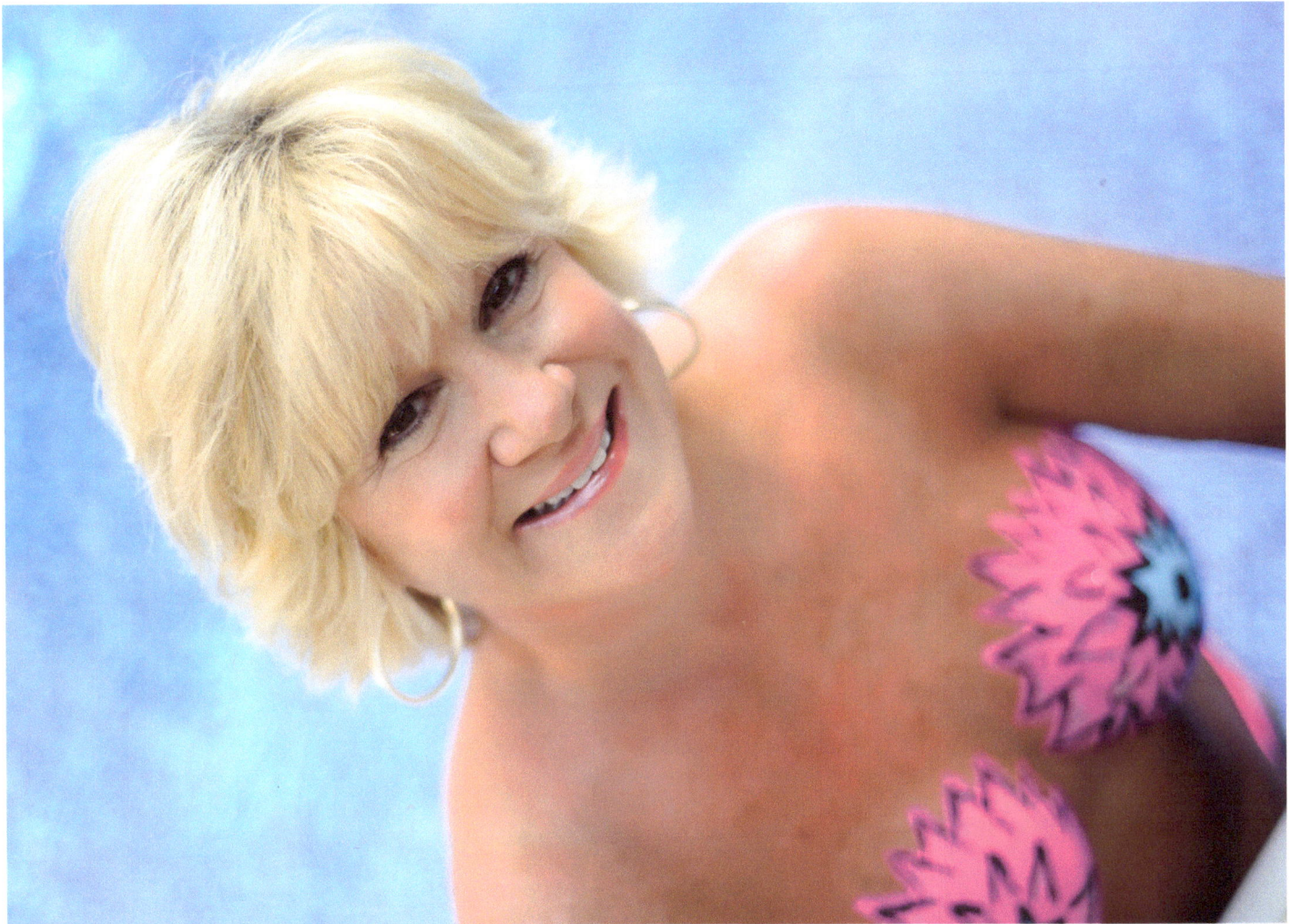

mend. They gave me several, mostly men. The office manager told me about a female plastic surgeon and said that everyone they had sent to her loved her. I decided she was the one for me and oh, was I so glad I did. On my first visit, she said, "I'll make you look better than before."

So, of course I was on board. I also made the decision to have a double mastectomy so I would not have to worry about this again.

Dr. Bouzaglou made all of the markings prior to surgery and today, you can barely even see my scars. The expanders were already in place when I awoke from my surgery. That is the real

"Thank goodness I learned about my options, including the option to see a plastic surgeon."

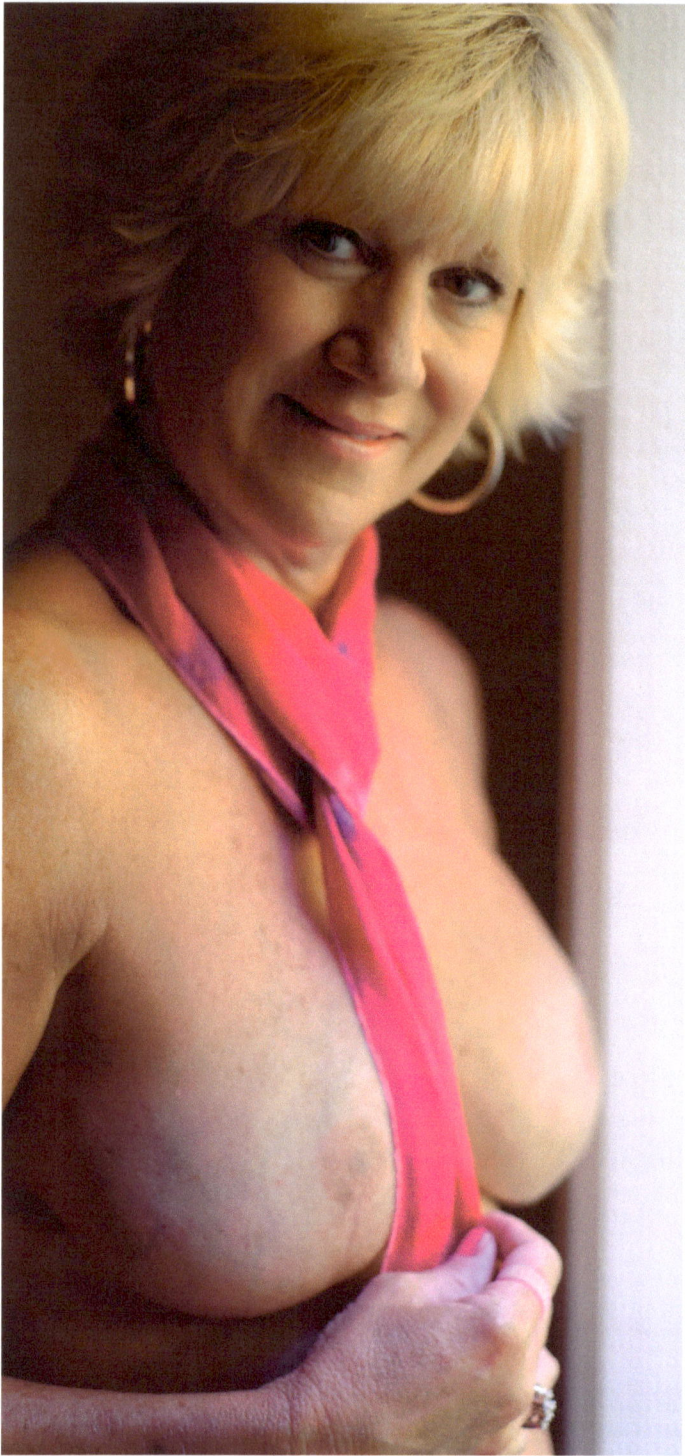

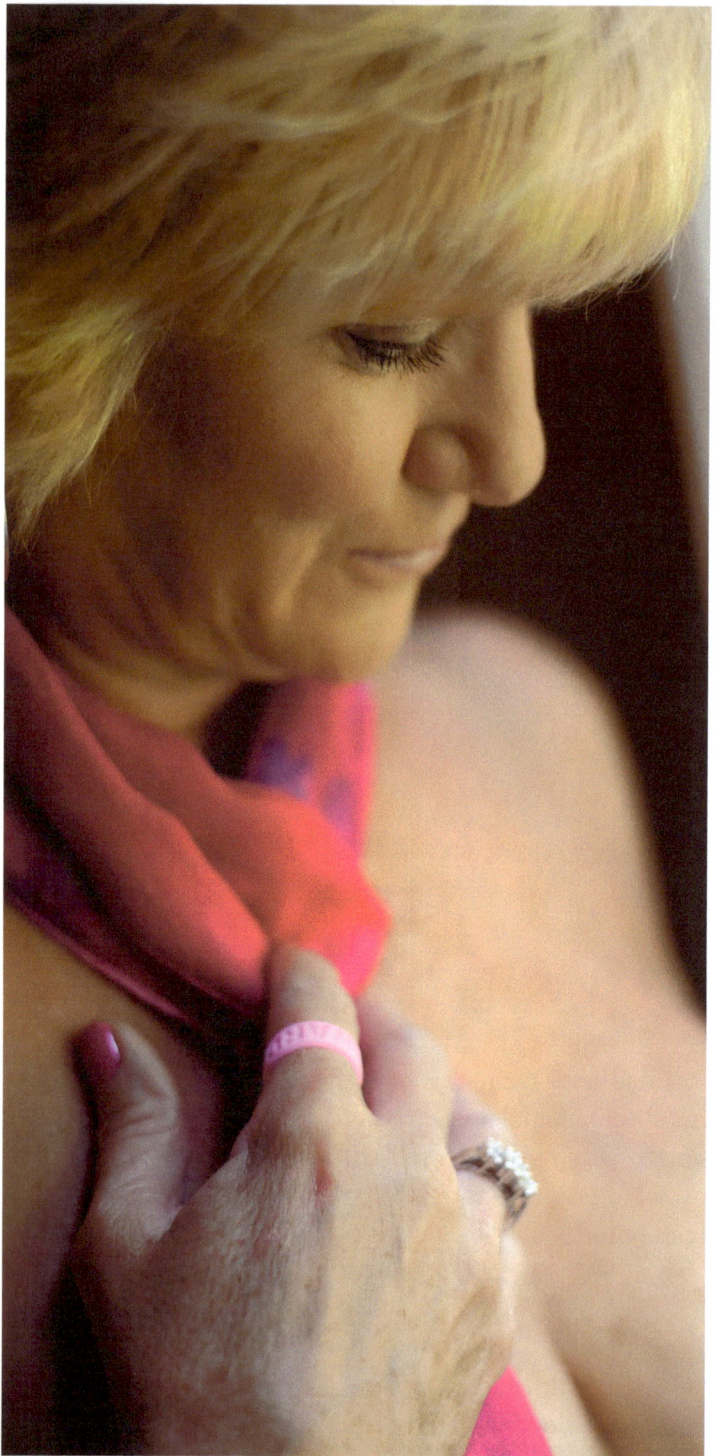

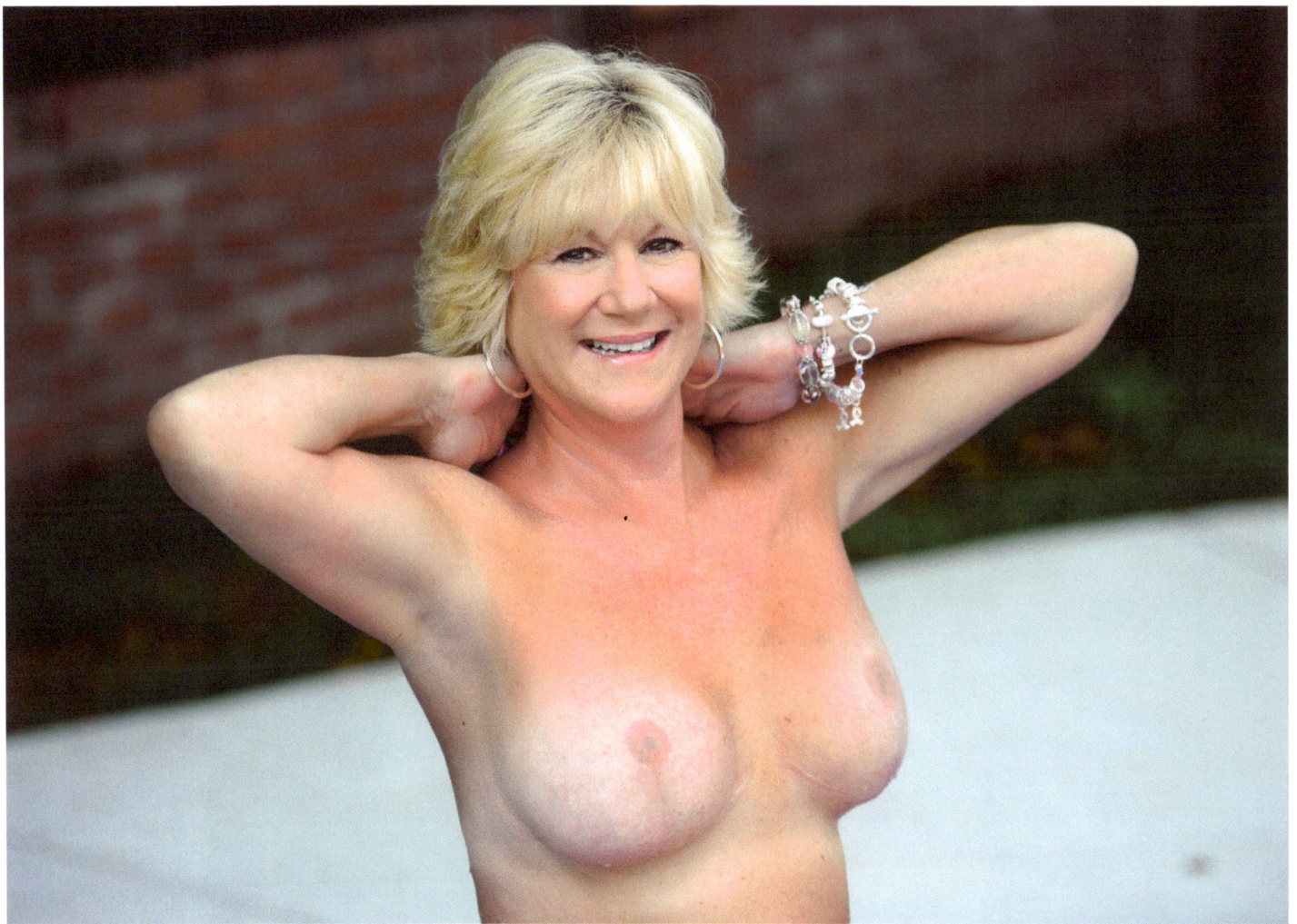

shocker, to wake up from something so scary and then to see that you already have some breasts again.

I went through the filling process, which is not bad at all. Then, I learned I needed to have four rounds of chemo as a precaution. That also turned out to be fine, I was not sick at anytime during this.

After finishing the chemo, I was ready for my permanent implants. Sure, it's not a walk in the park. I always hated the dreaded drains but I feel great and I think I look pretty good after all I have been through.

Thank God for plastic surgeons - especially mine!

Mary

My mother was diagnosed with breast cancer at sixty-two and had a mastectomy with no reconstruction. She is now eighty-one. My younger sister was diagnosed with breast cancer at forty-five. She had a lumpectomy followed by radiation and chemo. She was nearing her five-year survival point when I was diagnosed at the age of fifty-six.

Since my fortieth birthday, I'd been having annual mammograms with no problems. This time, I was called back in for a repeat.

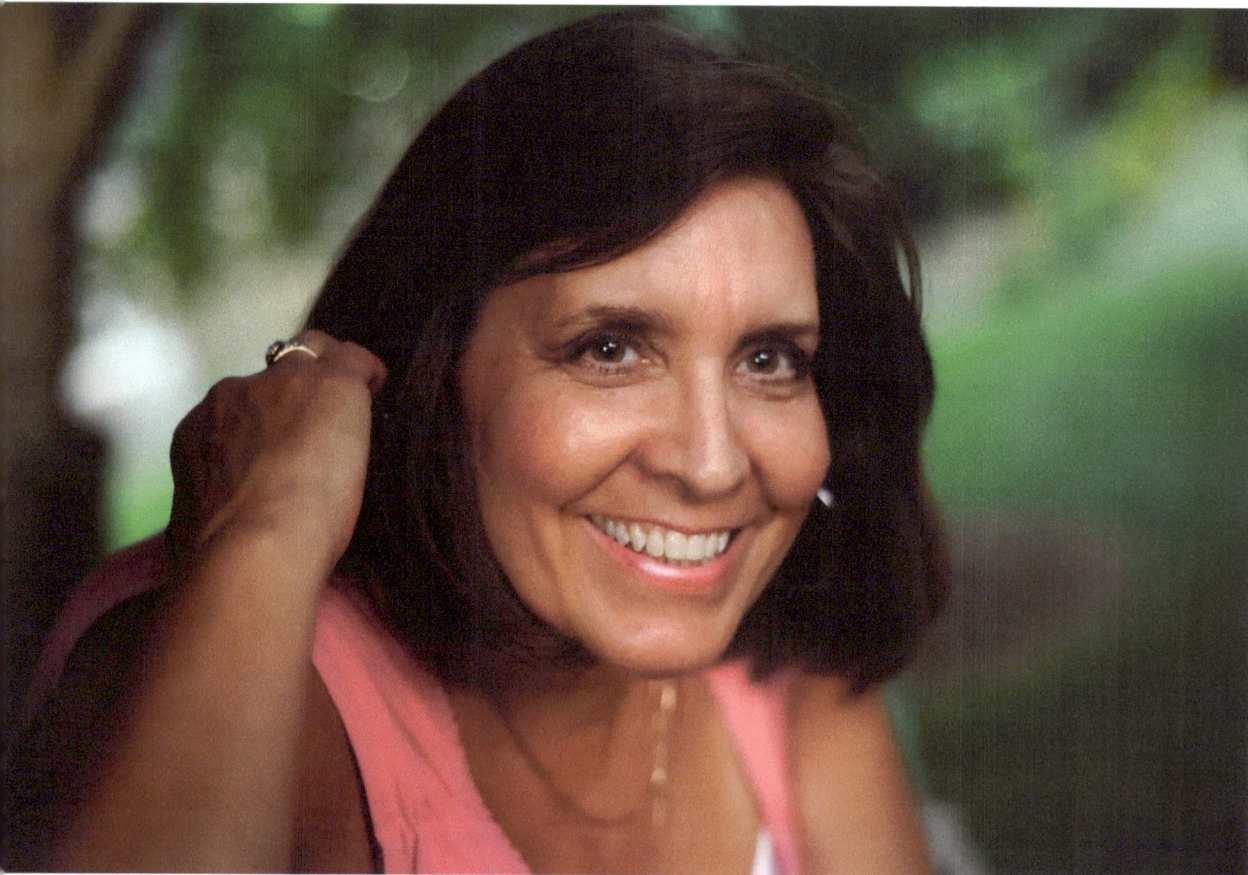

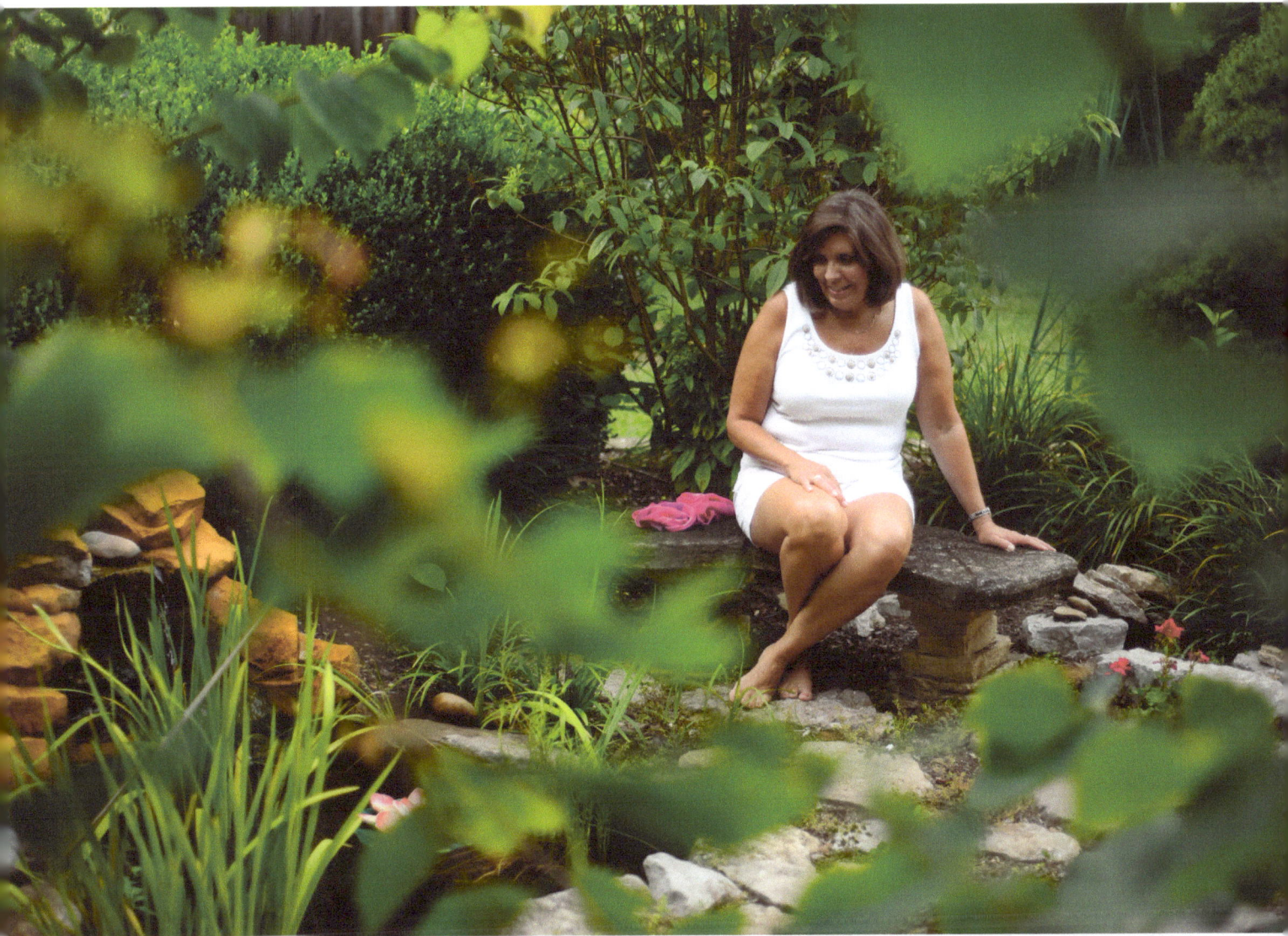

There were two areas in my left breast that were of concern, so a biopsy was recommended. The biopsies confirmed ductal carcinomas in both areas. The only foreign part of this news was that now it was me who had cancer.

Following my diagnosis, my husband, sister, and I met with a general surgeon, and we liked him. He spent ample time talking with us and communicated my situation and options well. He recommended a mastectomy and was open to consulting with a plastic surgeon about reconstruction. We scheduled the mastectomy to

"I am a private person, but I feel strongly that if my story can help even one woman who is facing breast cancer, then it's something I need to share."

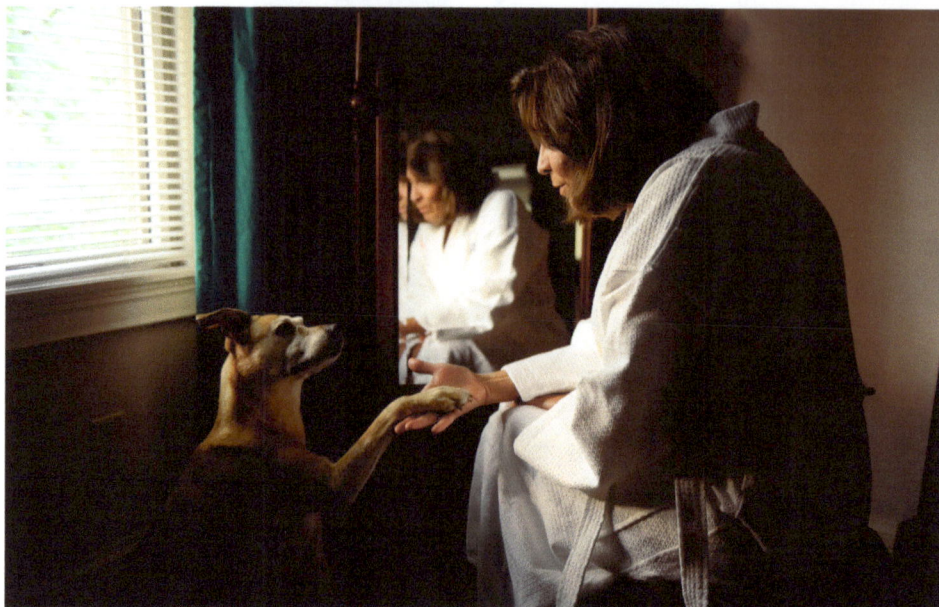

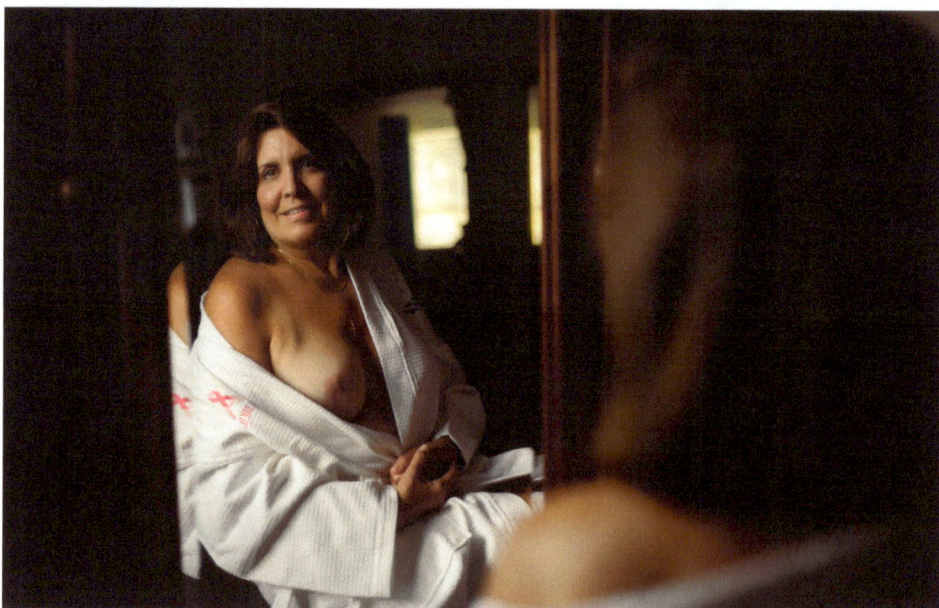

take place in three weeks, and his nurse made me an appointment to learn more about reconstruction.

We liked Dr. Bouzaglou immensely. Her enthusiasm and confidence made my decision simple. I found absolutely no reason not to have reconstruction. I had no previous health issues, no prescribed medications, etc., and I had a good insurance plan. Except for an absurdly high deductible, everything that I needed would be covered. That was a huge relief, a worry I did not have to bear.

I spent the two weeks before my surgery talking with the breast cancer survivors I knew. I reconnected with a childhood friend who'd had a mastectomy and reconstruction at age forty-five—eleven years earlier. My mom and sister were also survivors. They all shared their very personal experiences with me without hesitation.

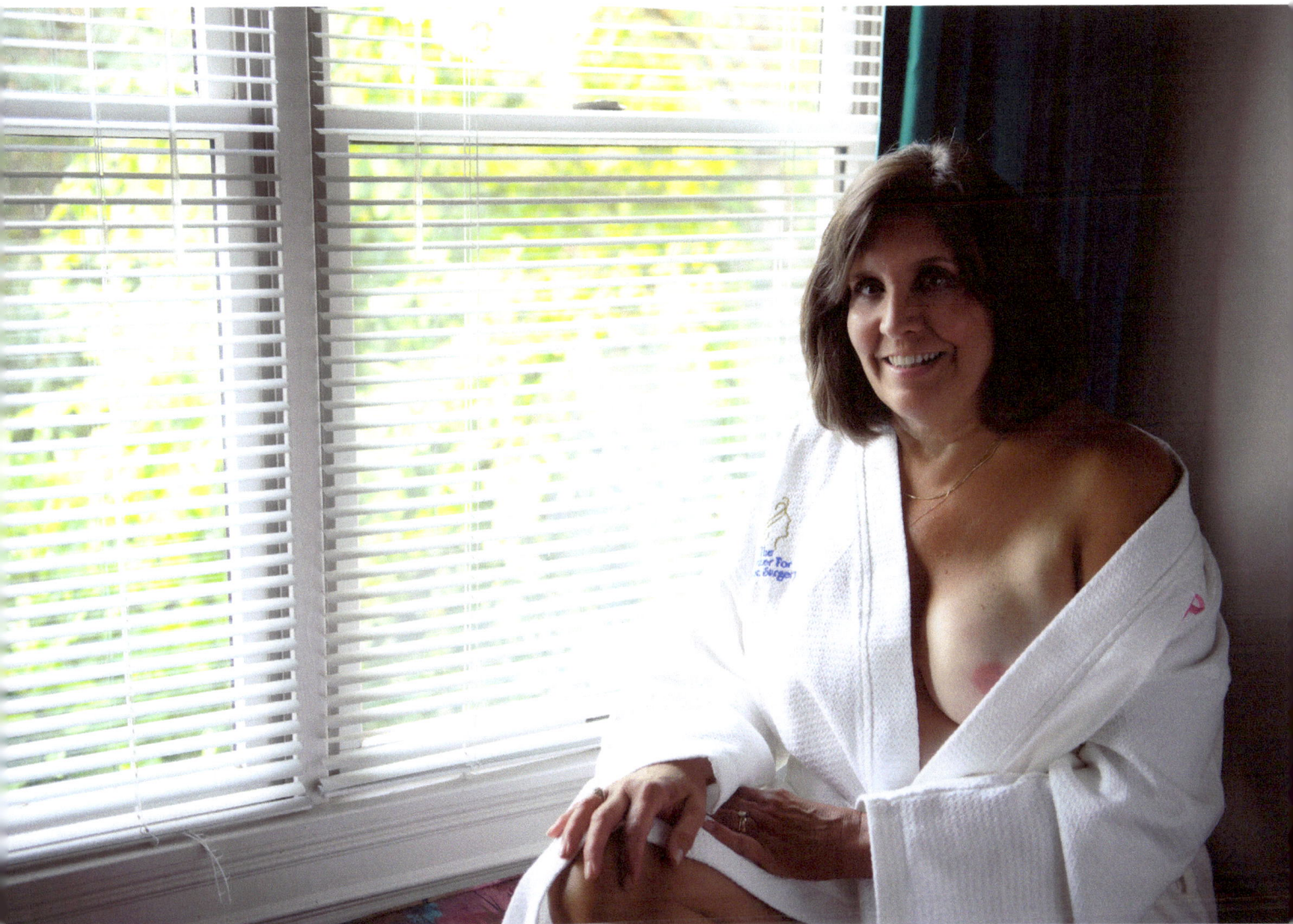

I didn't cry; I didn't feel sorry for myself; I was not afraid. But I did pray differently: I knew that no matter what God had for me, he would be with me. I recognized that he had been smoothing the path ahead of me, leading me to the best surgeons, and surrounding me with people who cared about me. I had never felt so loved.

Life around me didn't stop just because I had cancer. In fact, three weeks before my cancer diagnosis, my husband had been diagnosed with prostate cancer. He needed radiation but not

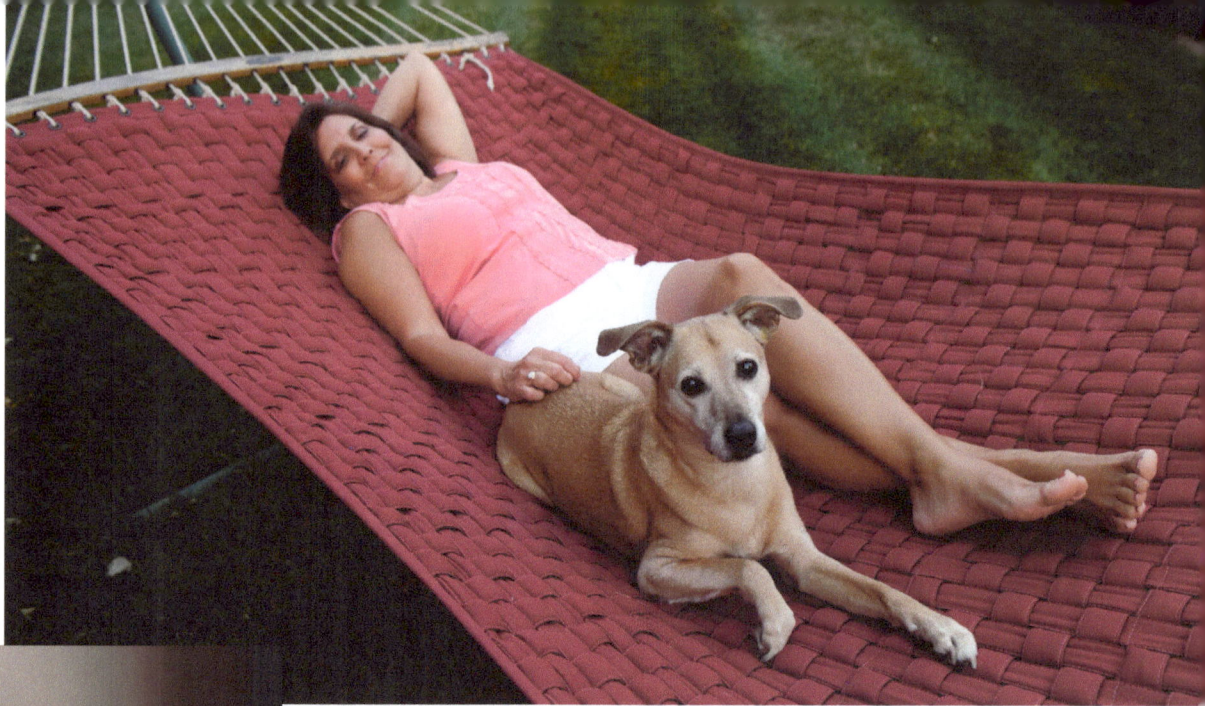

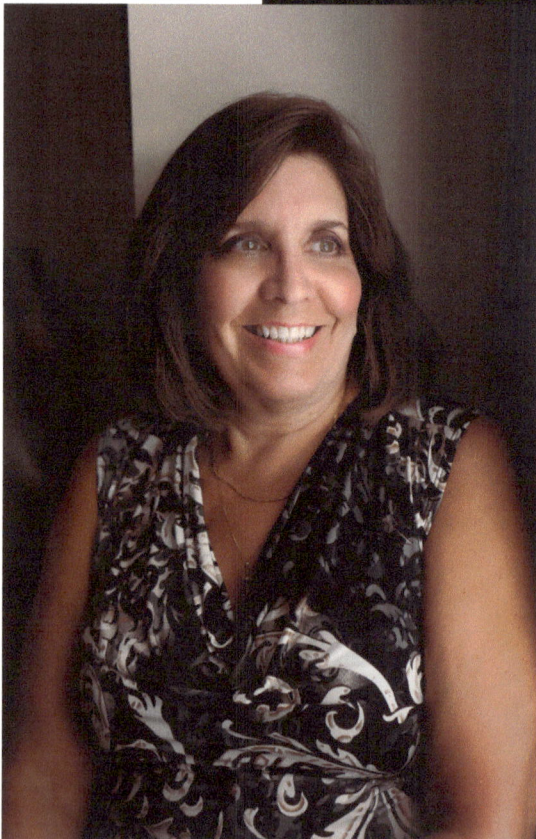

surgery. He received daily radiation treatments for nine weeks and was even able to get his treatment and see me the morning of my surgery. He promised to support whatever decision I made concerning reconstruction, and he has kept his word.

My sister lives eighty miles away, but she went with my husband and me to every consultation, every surgery, and even follow-up appointments. With her medical background, she asked questions that I had not considered. She and another sister spent the night at home with me before my surgery then stayed the next night in the hospital, taking care of me. I knew, too, on the morning of my surgery, that the women in my Bible study group were praying for me at that very time. It was very comforting.

My plastic surgeon began reconstruction immediately after my breast was removed by implanting a tissue expander. Final pathology reports determined that no chemo—and therefore no delay—would be necessary, so now I could get excited about my reconstruction. In time, the tissue expander was replaced with a permanent implant. Later, I had an implant and a lift done on my right breast so it would match the left. I had a tattoo done to replace the areola and then a fat injection, which included liposuction.

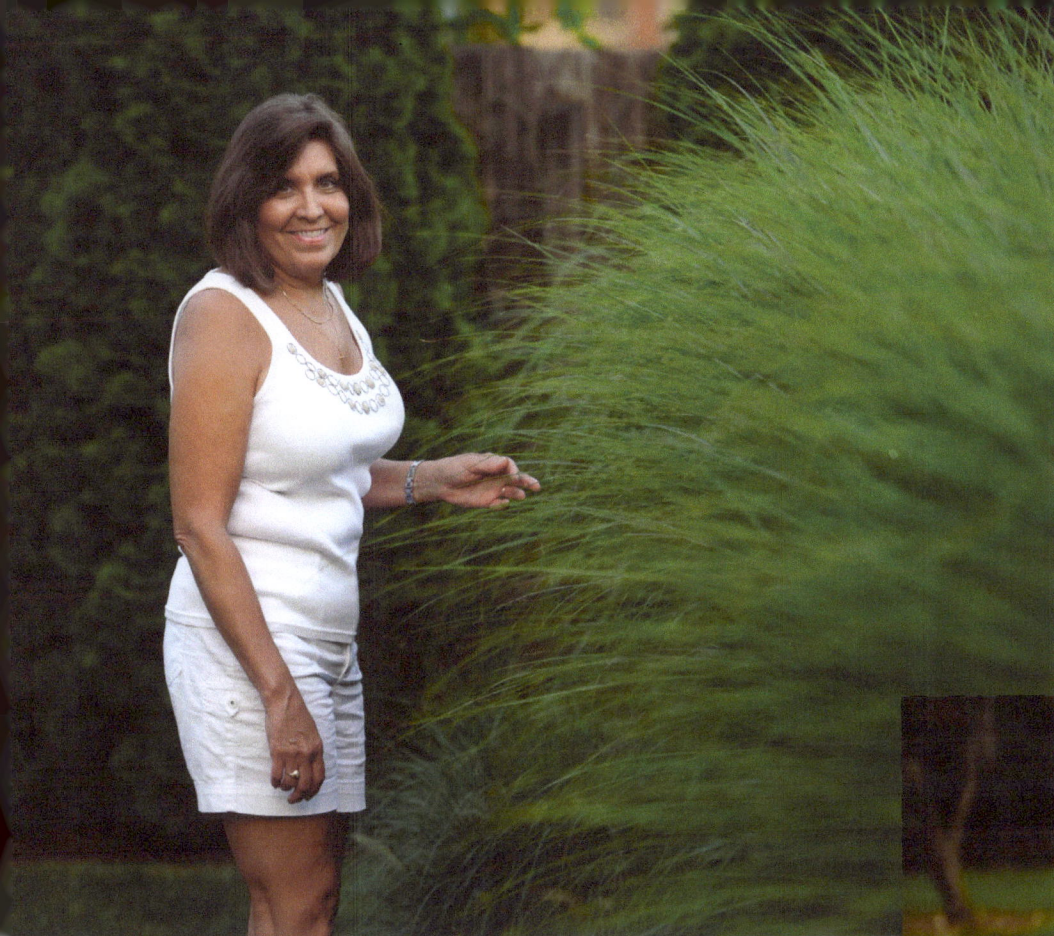

"I try to be much better about telling the people in my life that I love them and appreciate them."

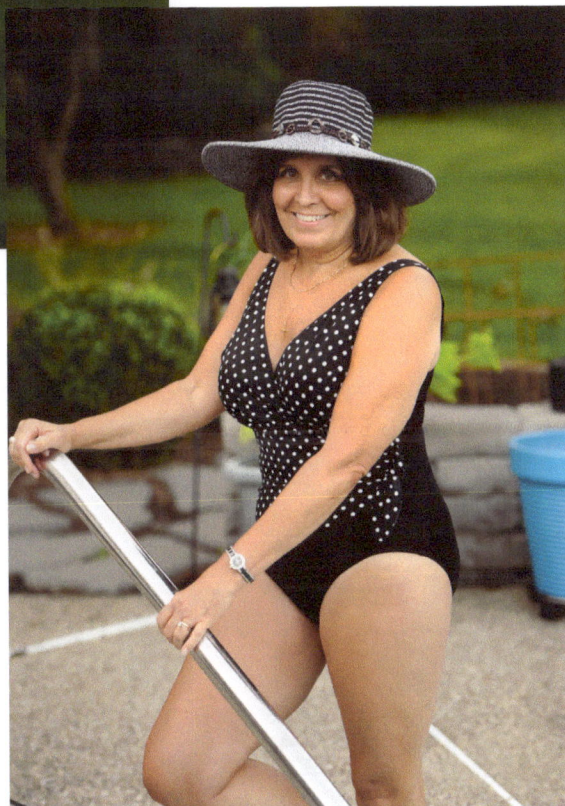

Despite all these surgeries and procedures, I had no post-op complications. There was much discomfort but little pain—pain pills took care of that. My healing progressed well. Through it all, I received incredible support, care, and faithful prayers from my family and friends. Because I chose faith over fear, my whole mastectomy/reconstruction experience was actually a peace-filled time for me. I try to be much better about telling the people in my life that I love them and appreciate them. I hope I am a better person.

I am a private person, but I feel strongly that if my story can help even one woman who is facing breast cancer, then it's something I need to share. I am completely satisfied with the results of my breast reconstruction. I can wear the clothes I like and even forget that I ever had cancer. Gene testing has been mentioned as something I might consider, but as of now I am undecided.

Lisa

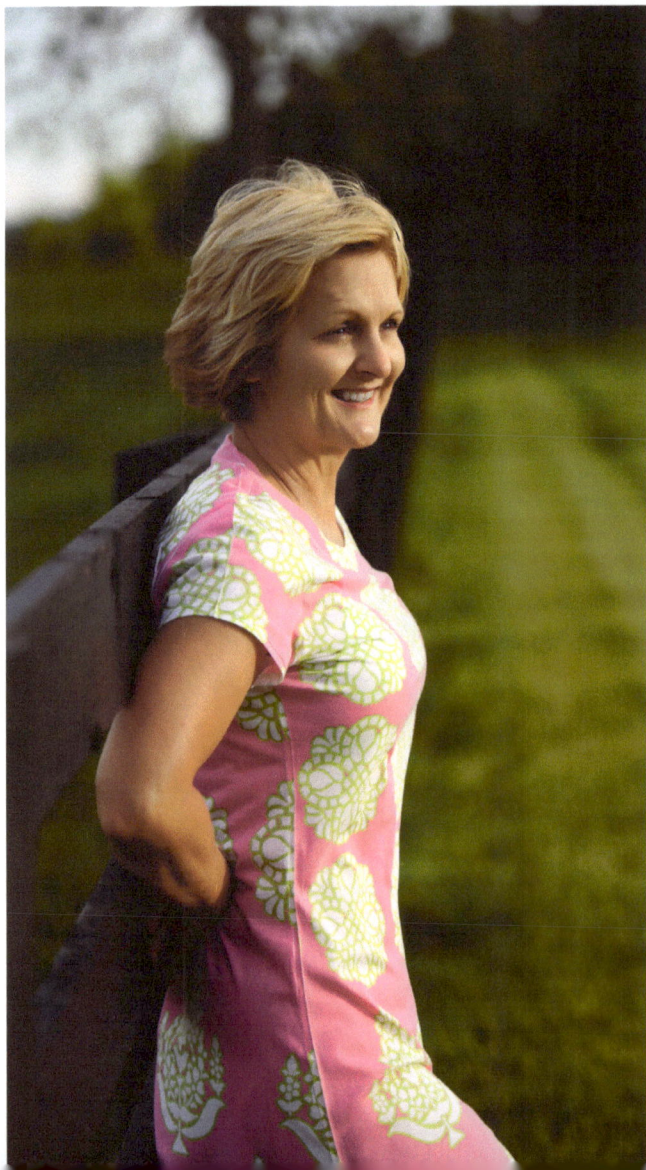

Cancer—the dreaded word no one wants to hear.

Unfortunately, my family has been dealing with cancer since 1998. My children have spent half their lives with cancer in front of them. It started when my husband, Mike, was diagnosed with non-Hodgkin's lymphoma in 1998. He went through chemotherapy and then a stem cell transplant in 1999. During the summer of 2006, he contracted a virus, which led to a trip to the ER, where they discovered his blood counts were low. Further testing revealed that he had myelodysplastic syndrome, a side effect of the radiation he'd received during his transplant. He was scheduled for a nonrelated-donor bone marrow transplant in October 2006.

Mike came through the transplant fine but developed secondary infections by November. His kidneys shut down from graft-versus-host disease, and he contracted CMV, both of which should have been fatal. Again, he pulled through. The doctors and nurses started calling him the "comeback kid."

Nine more weeks in the hospital physically weakened him to the point that he required a month's rehabilitation. He still faced problems with his kidneys and bladder from the graft–versus-host disease, but he kept making progress. During his recovery, our daughter was married, and he actu-

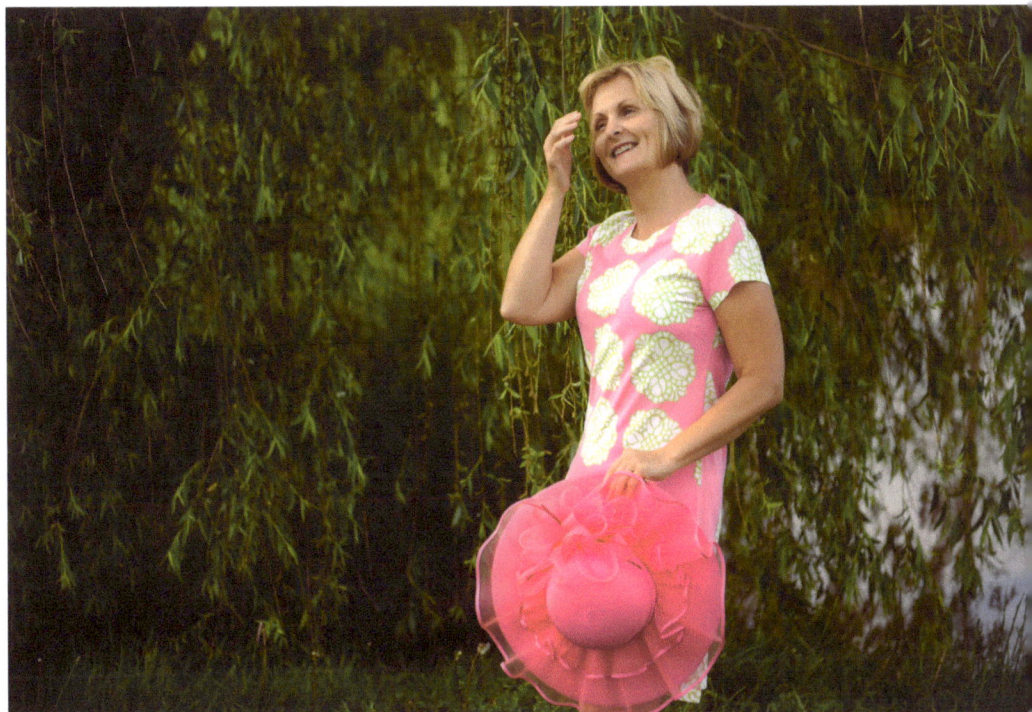

ally walked her down the aisle. It was such a wonderful day for us.

The fall of 2007 brought more recovery. During this time, I consulted with a plastic surgeon for a breast reduction, something I had wanted for a while but had not done because of Mike's recovery. I scheduled the surgery for late December.

Mike was progressing so well that we decided to go to a friend's house in Florida for Thanksgiving. While we were there, Mike developed pneumonia and became septic. He was admitted to the hospital in Florida and we remained there for three weeks. Finally, we were flown home on a medevac jet, and he was admitted to the ICU.

I kept in touch with my plastic surgeon so I could keep my surgery date of December 28. My children would be home for Christmas, and I knew they would help out with their dad and everything would be okay. But Mike's health continued to deteriorate, and he passed away on December 21.

I called the office and the surgeon suggested I postpone the surgery due to my mental state, but something just kept telling me to go through with it. My children would be home through Christmas and able to help. If I waited, I would be home alone and probably put the surgery off for a while or not have it at all. So I kept my surgery scheduled for December 28, the day after Mike's funeral.

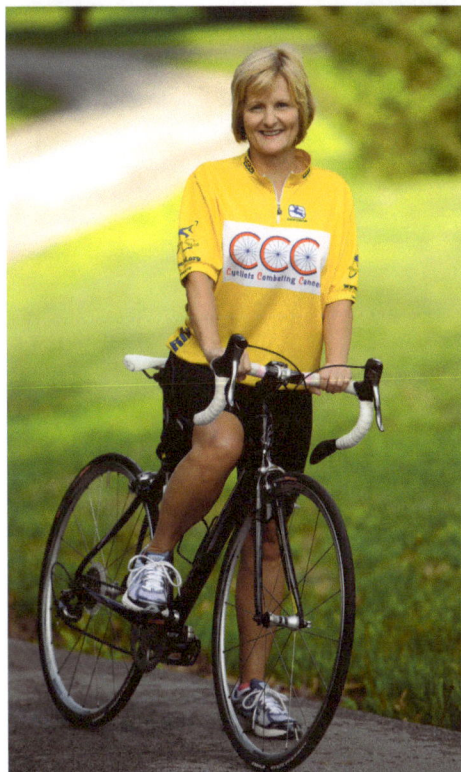

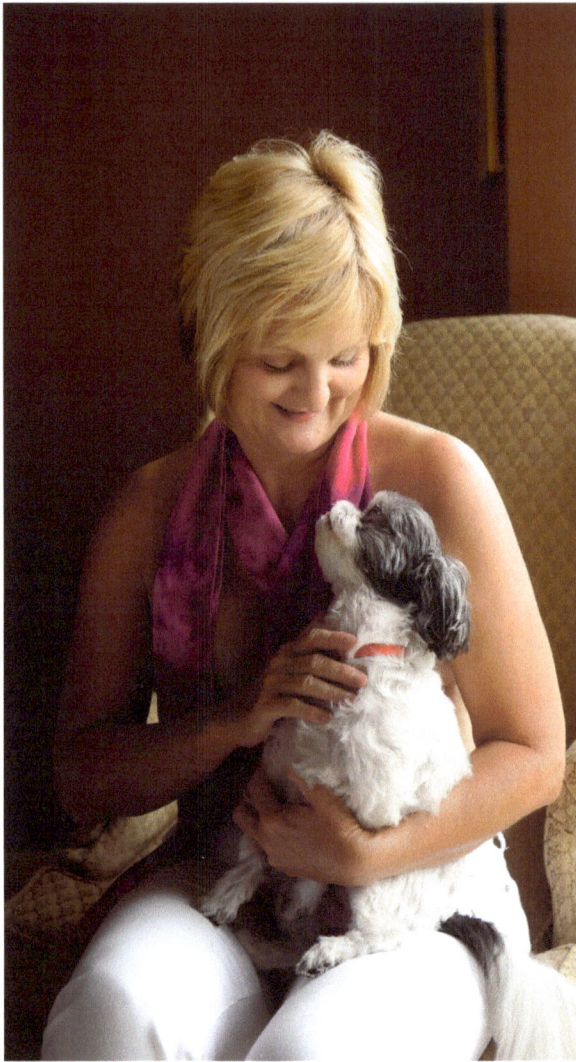

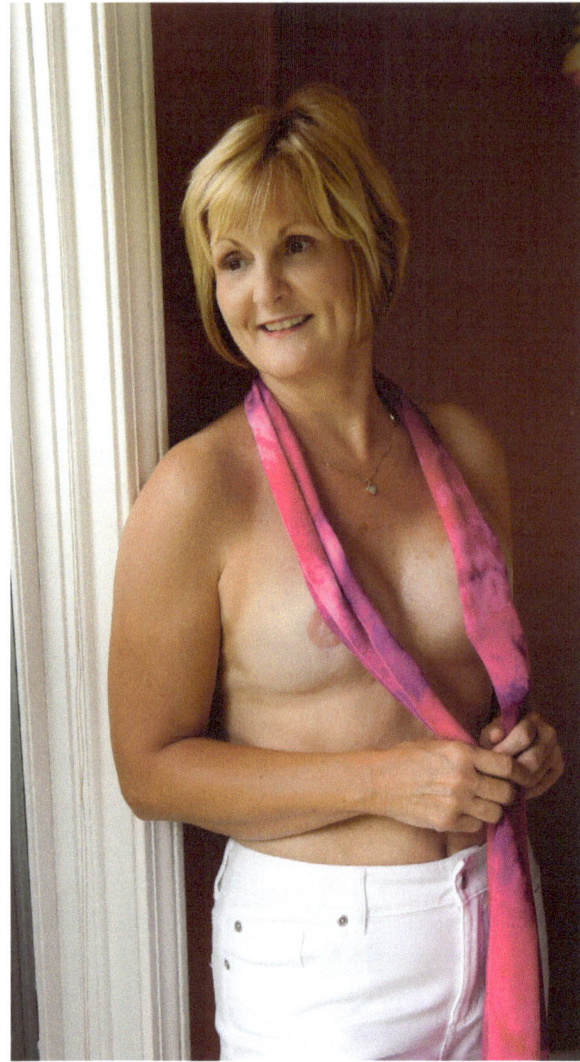

I am so thankful that I did.

The surgery went great. I felt fine except the mental numbness from Mike's death. Then ten days later, the plastic surgeon called with some news. She told me that the pathologist had found a ductal carcinoma in one of my breasts and that I needed to see a surgeon.

I couldn't even comprehend what she was telling me. I just thanked her and hung up the phone. My daughter was there and wanted to know what the call was about. The plastic surgeon had called three days earlier to check on my healing, so my daughter thought it was unusual to get another call so soon.

I told her, "I don't know, something about a carcinoma." I

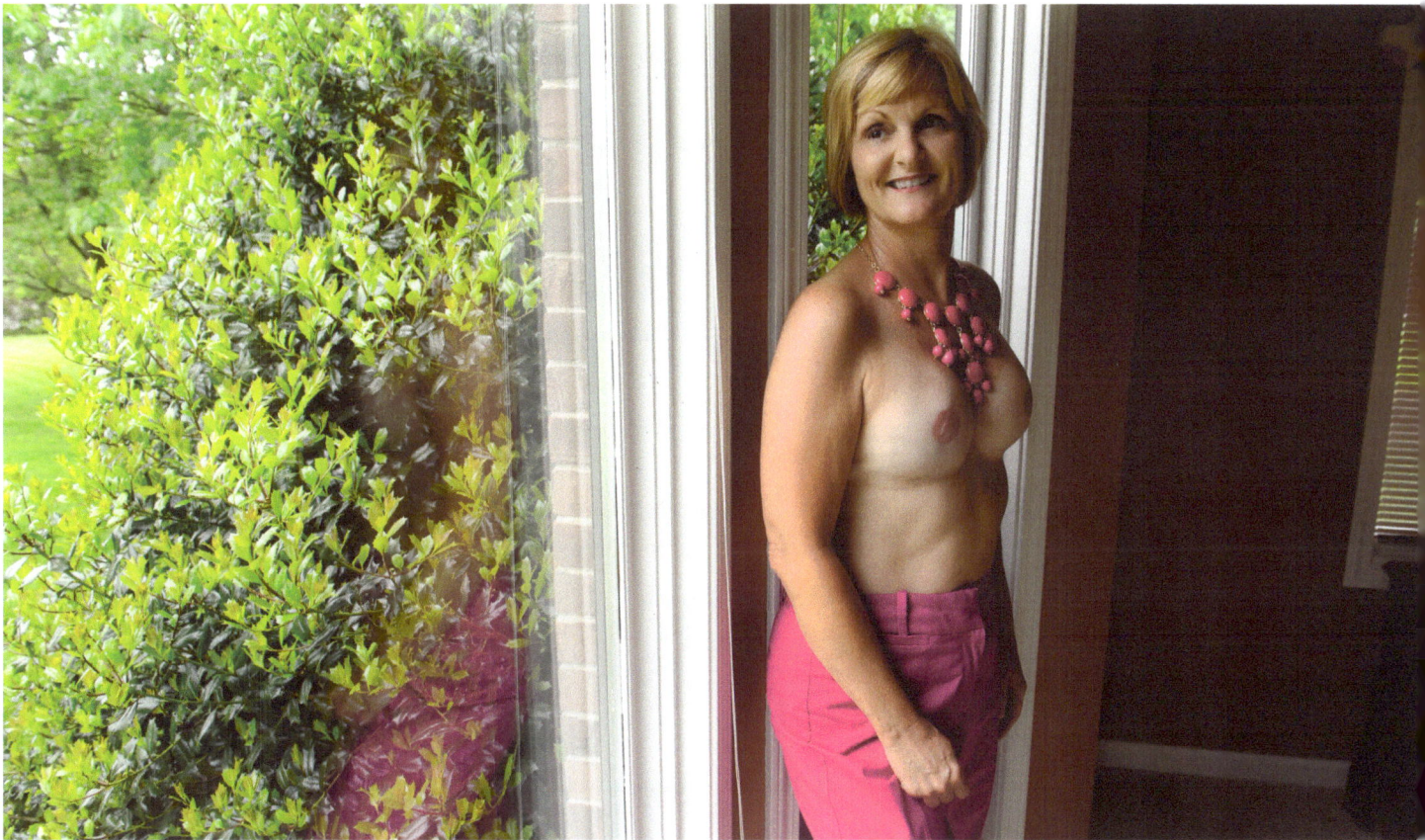

couldn't even think what the surgeon had told me. Quickly, I returned her call and asked her to repeat what she had just said. The plastic surgeon gave me the information again, as well as the name and phone numbers of a general surgeon.

My mind was reeling. How was this possible? I'd had a mammogram during my pre-op, and nothing had shown up. Was I one of the statistics where cancer is found that hadn't shown on the mammogram? So many questions.

My support group during Mike's illness and death included two dear friends who are physicians. I immediately called them and told them the news. They got me scheduled with a surgeon within a week. At my scheduled appointment, the medical team reviewed

"It's really not about how they look, though, because nobody sees them but me. It's about the way I feel."

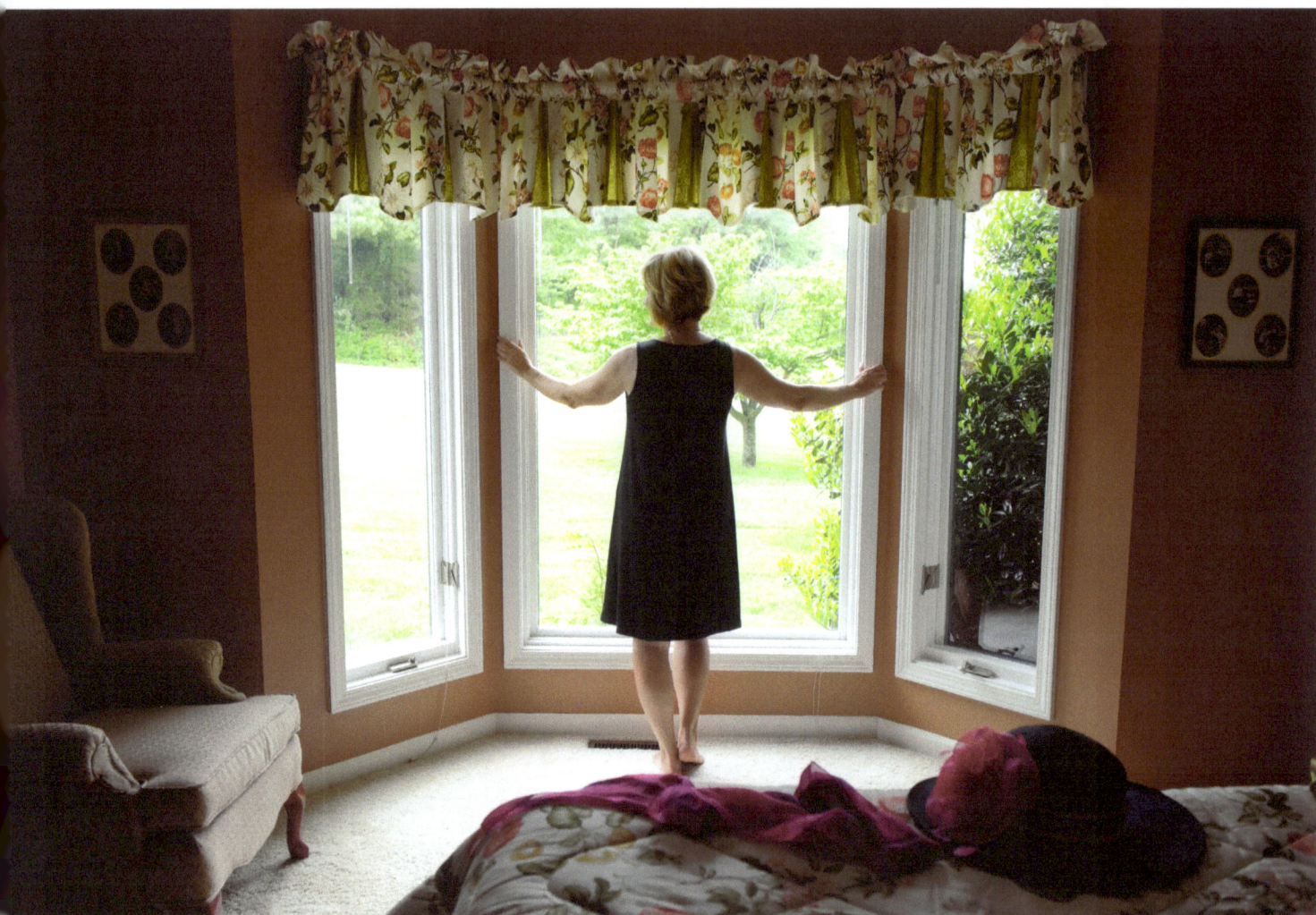

my information and came back with two recommendations—either a mammogram every three weeks to follow the carcinoma or a bilateral mastectomy with possible radiation or chemotherapy. I knew the answer immediately—a bilateral mastectomy. My children, though they were twenty-one and twenty-four, couldn't take any more stress and worry in their lives.

I consulted with my plastic surgeon about breast reconstruction. She and my general surgeon coordinated the surgery: a bilateral mastectomy followed by the start of breast reconstruction.

> *"In fact, a lot of people would never know that I have faced breast cancer."*

Luckily, I did not need radiation or chemotherapy.

The reconstruction experience went well. My plastic surgeon harvested the nipple from the breast that was not involved and placed it on my abdomen for use during the reconstruction. The tissue expanders were filled to the desired breast size, the implants were placed, and finally the nipple transferred and sculpted into two.

Sometimes, I forget that I have gone through all of this because of how good my reconstruction looks. It's really not about how they look, though, because nobody sees them but me. It's about the way I feel. I still feel whole. I don't worry about how my clothes fit or if I can wear a low-cut top, and I don't worry about using a prosthesis. In fact, a lot of people would never know that I have faced breast cancer.

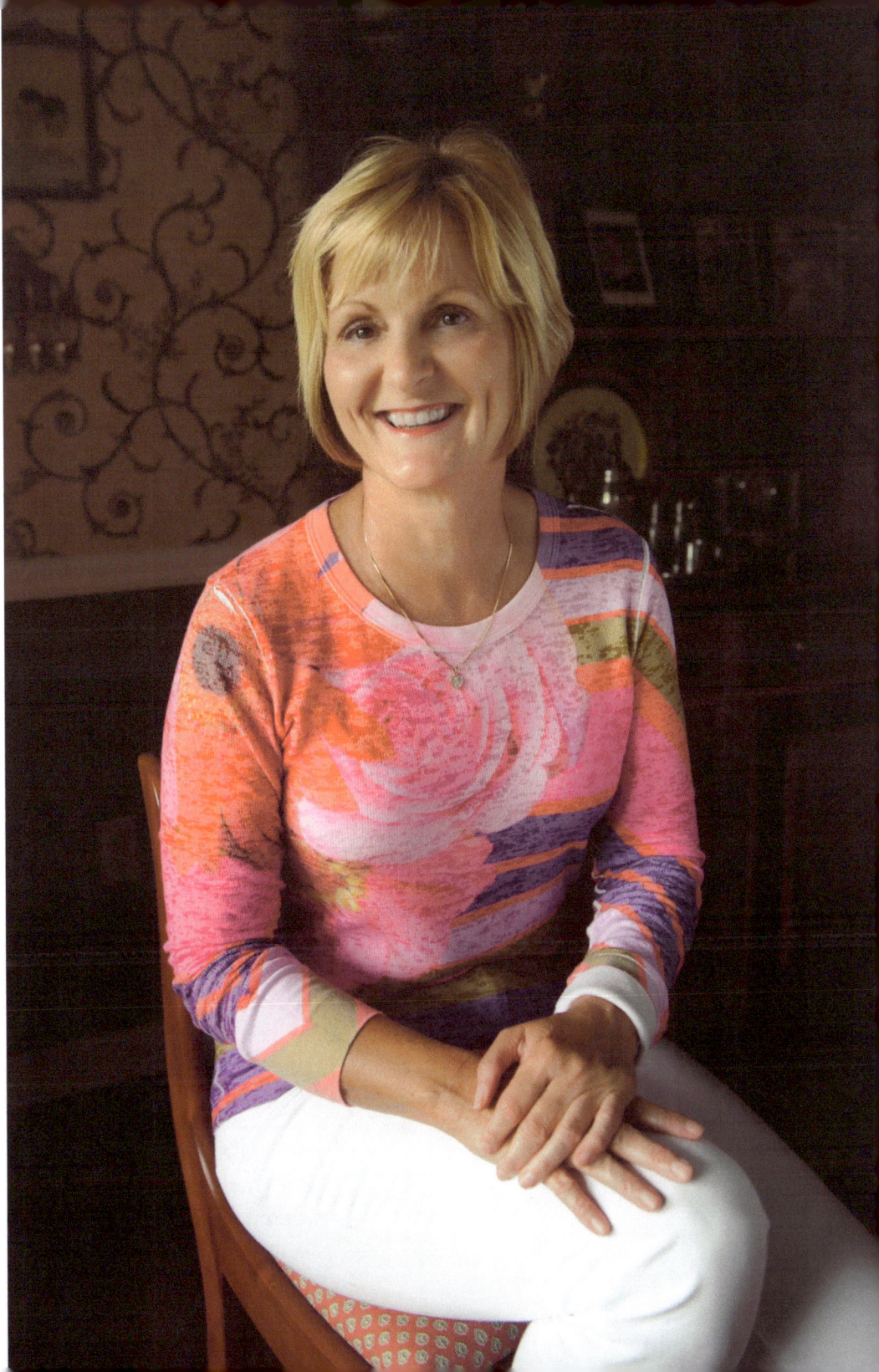

Susan

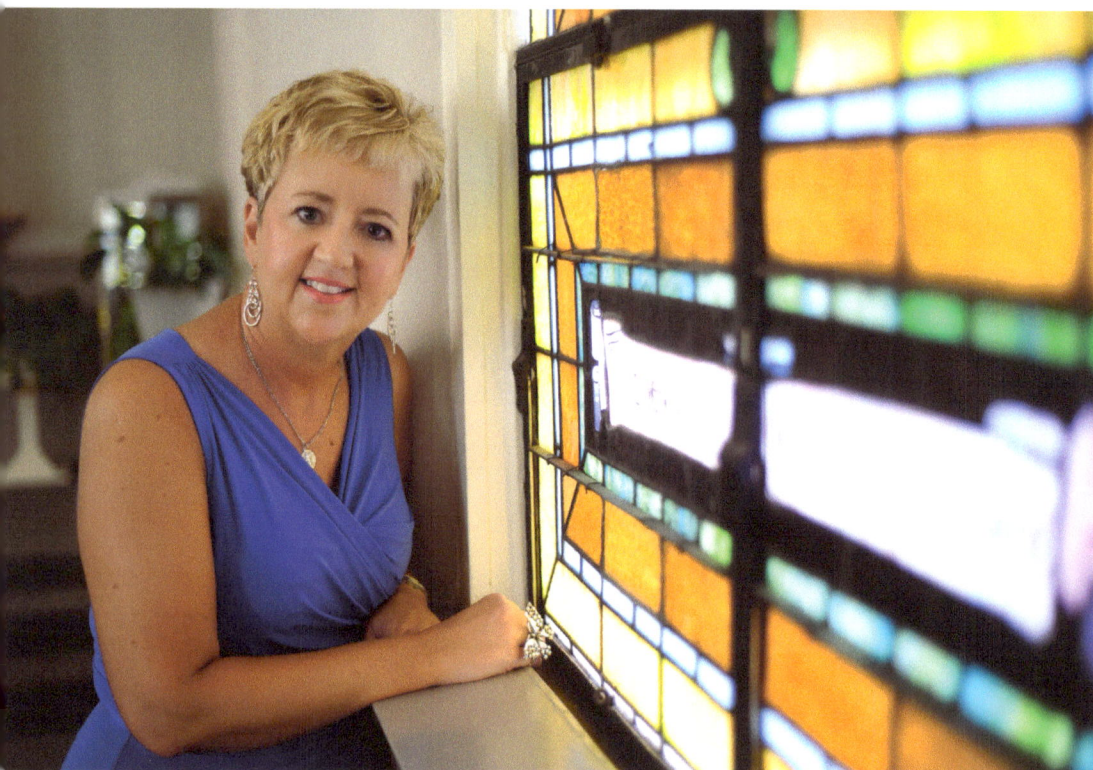

Do you remember where you were when you found out about the terrorist attack on the twin towers on 9/11?

Every woman who has had breast cancer remembers when and where she was when she found out she had the dreaded disease. She realizes that her life will never be the same.

My name is Susan and I was getting ready to teach a Zumba class on May 25th, 2012 when I got the call. Everything in me went numb and all the details were lost.

"You have cancer," was all I heard.

But let me go back a little further and tell you a little about me.

I married very young, at the age of seventeen, and am still married. I had my first blessing, a son, that same year. Twelve years later, my daughter came along. Throughout their childhood, I worked a full-time job and did all the things that working moms do, looking forward to the time that I could retire and do the things

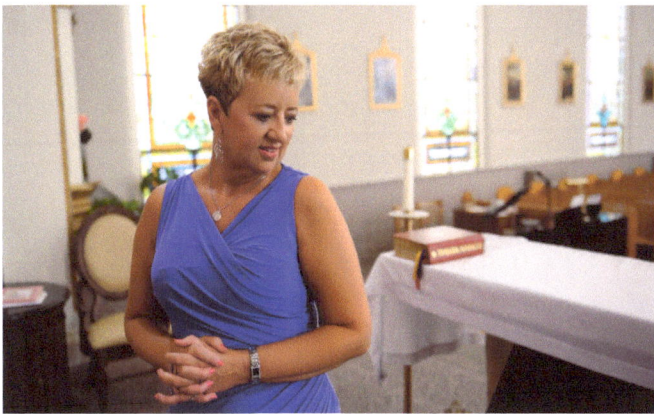

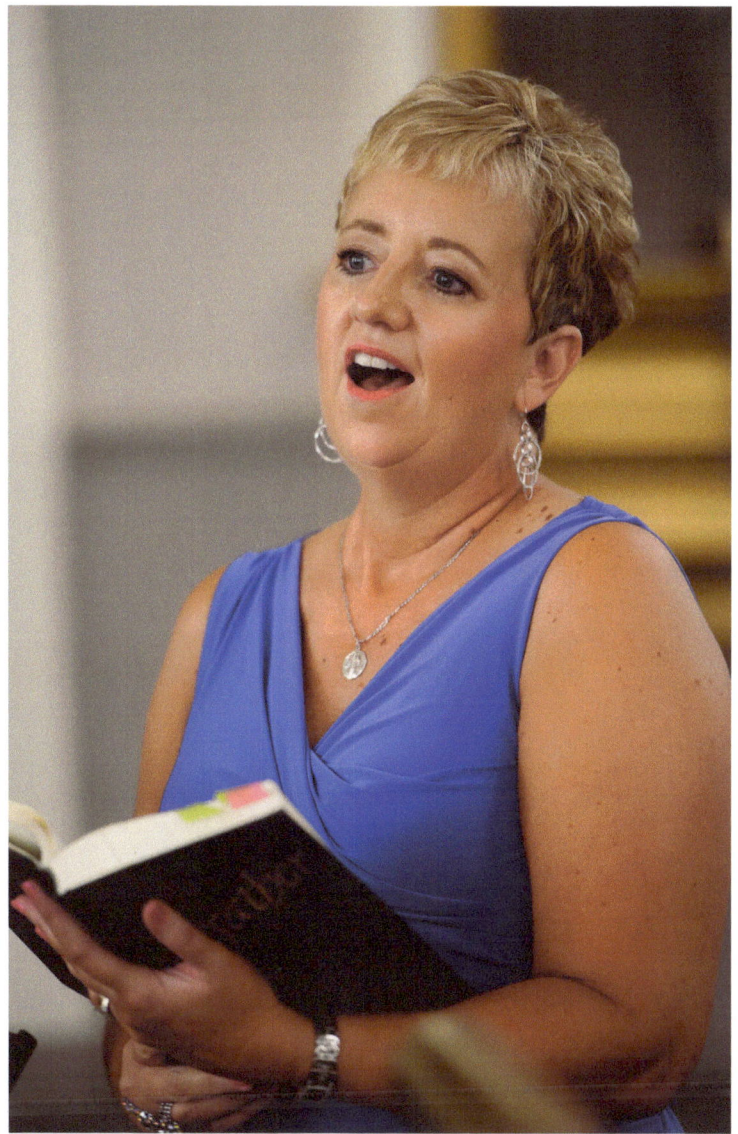

I wanted to do.

I retired on July 1st, 2011, after twenty-three years at a utility company. Suddenly, it was my time. I enjoyed traveling (especially to the beach), teaching Zumba classes, reading, singing with choirs, spending time on Facebook and doing what I wanted to do.

The first time I had a mammogram, somewhere around the age of forty, they called me back for an ultrasound and I was concerned I might have cancer. In the years that followed, every time I went for my mammogram, I needed more tests (more mammograms, ultra-sounds, aspirations, biopsies). I was told that I had very "dense" breast tissue, as well as fibro tumors that had to be aspirated when the cysts got uncomfortable. I had several biopsies done.

In September 2010, I even had a lumpectomy that came back negative for cancer. Since my mother had breast cancer when she was sixty-nine, I also decided to have the BRACA gene testing done. This also came back negative.

After this round of testing, I felt very relieved. I let myself relax a little, knowing I wouldn't have to be checked again for a while. I retired and got on with enjoying my life of not sitting behind a desk for eight hours a day.

In October 2011, it was time for another mammogram. I put it off, dreading the tests I knew they would put me through. Dreading the metal table I would have to lie on, while my breasts

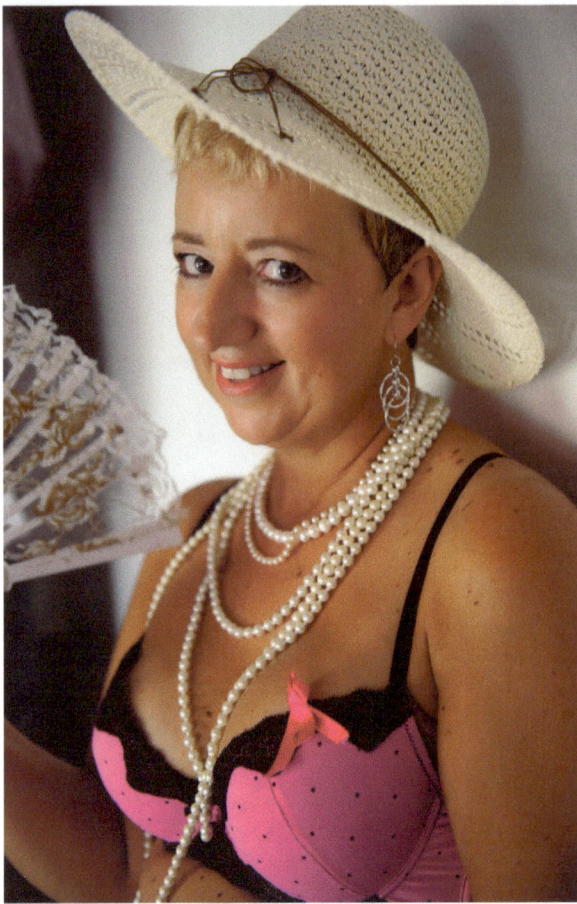

"No one knows what tomorrow will bring. So, I want to feel confident and happy with my body."

hung underneath me and got poked and picked at. Finally, after my husband urged me to have one of the cysts checked out, I made an appointment for a diagnostic mammogram on May 24th, 2012.

I had the mammogram, ultra-sound and biopsy done all the same day. I received a call with the bad news the next day. Curiously, the cancer was not in the breast that had the cyst in it, but the other one.

I decided to have a bi-lateral mastectomy so that I wouldn't be worried about the other breast the rest of my life. No more mammograms!!

As I said before, I enjoyed being on Facebook when I retired and made many new friends. One of them, Genea, was battling breast cancer. I followed her journey. She had lots of support and seemed to be handling it very well.

Genea was the first person I called when I got the news. I was in shock and didn't even know how to tell anyone. She dropped what she was doing and came to my house immediately.

I will never forget it: Genea made me see that everything was going to be all right. She even offered to show me what she looked like after her surgery. I was amazed! She looked good!

Now, I was thinking that maybe I could look even better than before. Because she had done so well and looked so good, I decided to use both her surgeon and plastic surgeon.

Genea also helped me with my hair. My hair has always been one of my best assets. It is very thick and was naturally blonde well into my thirties. The majority of the time, during chemo, most of your hair falls out. I wanted to be prepared, so Genea went with

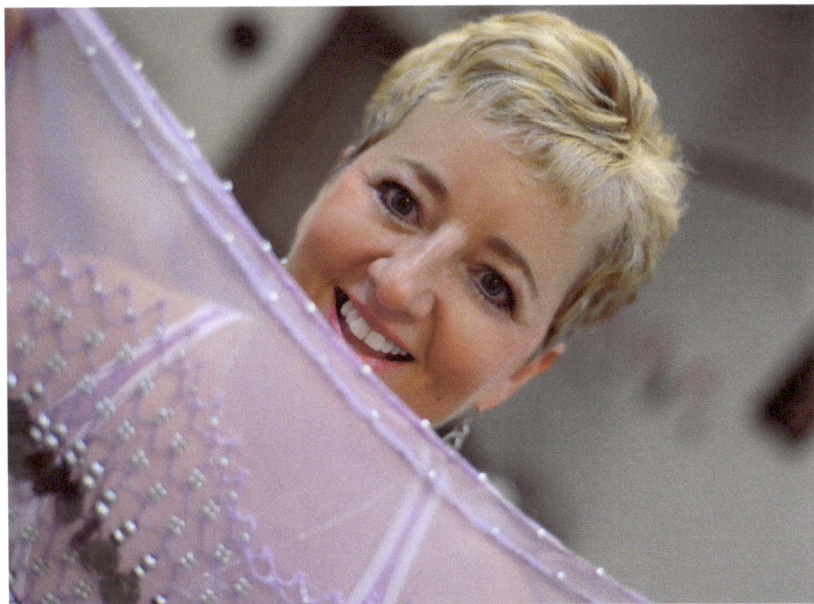

me to pick out wigs. When the time came to have my hair shaved off, she was there with a hat and scarf for me to wear. Afterwards, she took me for a ride in her convertible. I often tell her she is an angel that God sent to me to help me get through this.

On February 7th, 2012, I finished my chemo. Interestingly, my hair has come back in very curly.

My breast reconstruction is almost complete. I just have to have a couple more small adjustments to make them look as good as new. I think that after it is all done, I will look just about the same as before, except for the scar from under my nipple down. In time, that will get less noticeable.

Why should I worry about having pretty breasts when I am fifty years old and happily married?

The answer is this: we never know how long we have to live. We could walk out the door tomorrow and be struck by lightning! We have to live as though we will live to be one hundred. No one knows what tomorrow will bring. So, I want to feel confident and happy with my body.

I'm not teaching Zumba again yet, but I am going to classes and getting back into shape. One night at class, my instructor told me about a friend of hers that had been diagnosed with breast cancer. This was a Monday and she was having surgery on Friday, just

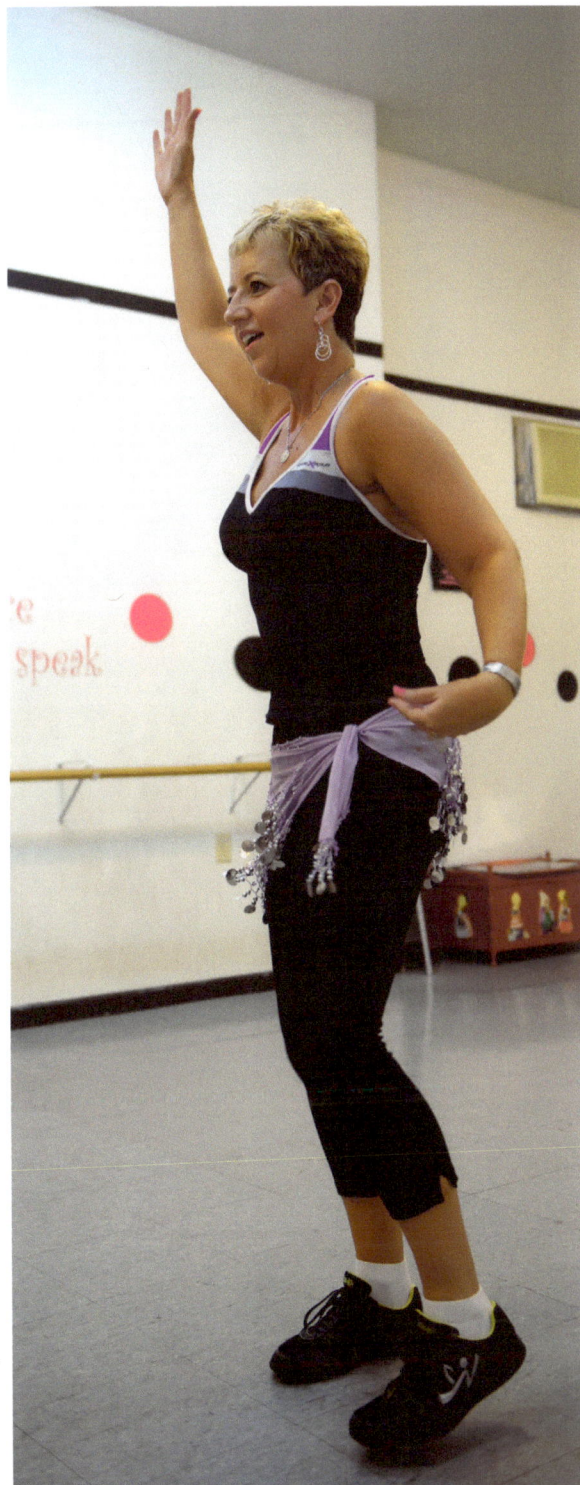

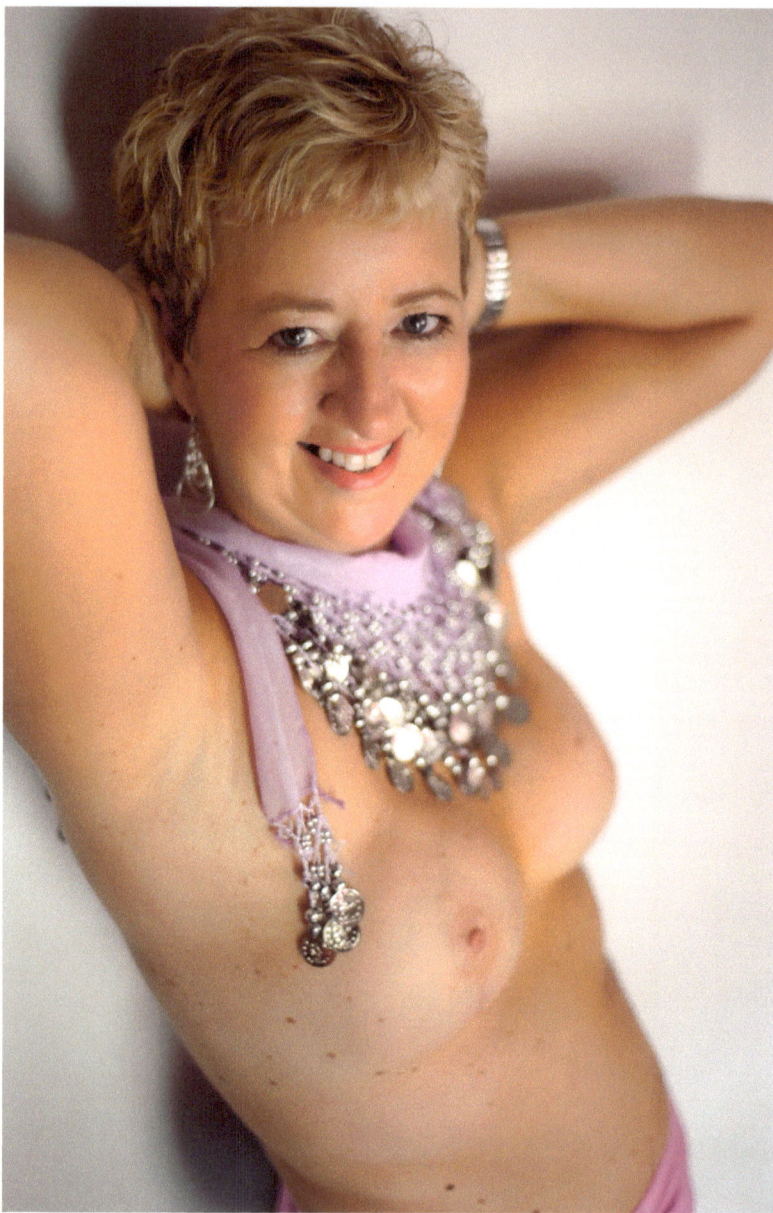

"your life can be normal again."

four days later.

I told my instructor to have her friend call me. I wanted to know if she was having the skin saving type of mastectomy as well. When we spoke, I learned her surgeon had not even mentioned this to her.

She got on the phone the next day and found a plastic surgeon to work with her general surgeon on that short notice. Her general surgeon called, wanting to know why she was doing this! She told him that it would save her another surgery and she could tell he wasn't happy about it.

I want to get the word out to every woman who may be going through this that your life can be normal again. It's a new kind of normal. No, your breasts aren't going to look exactly the same as they did before. But I have found a lot of positive things have happened to me since I have been diagnosed with cancer.

You may find that your spouse is more romantic and caring than you ever thought. You may be surprised by how many people consider themselves your friend and shower you with gifts, cards, food and prayers. I was.

Everyone said to me "You have such a good attitude." I think my faith in God has helped me as much as anything else. I am not afraid to die, because I do believe in heaven and I believe

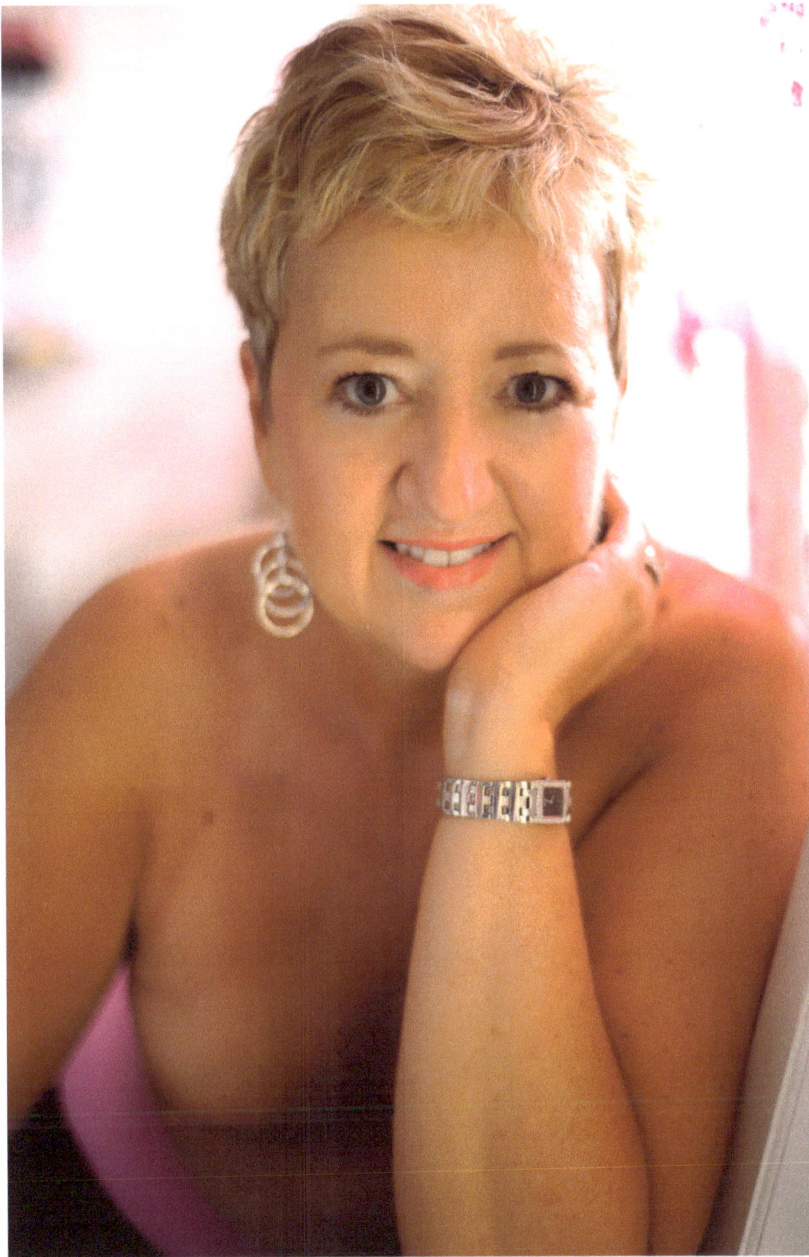

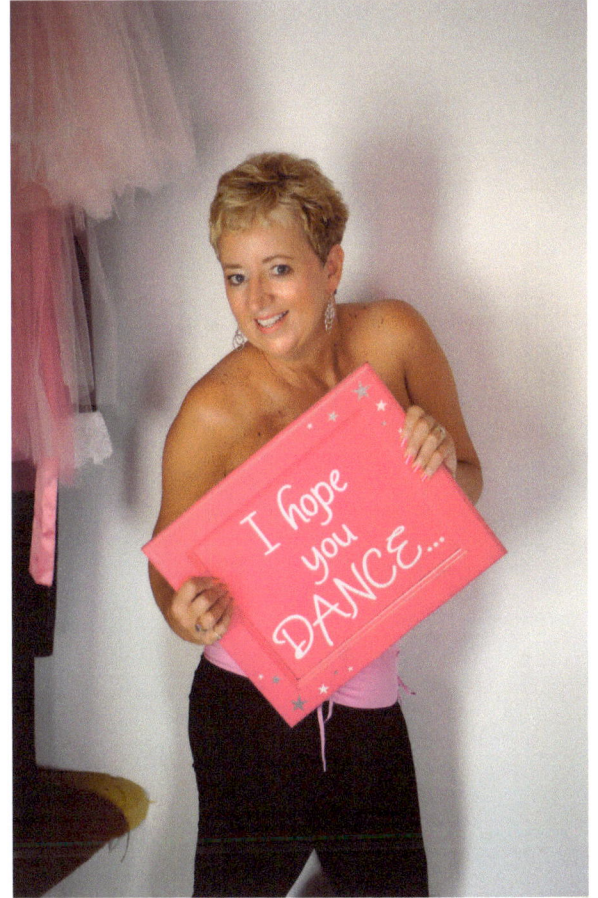

I will be there some day.

My favorite quote is: "Lord I know that you will not give me more than I can handle, I just wish you wouldn't trust me so much!" - Mother Teresa of Calcutta

Lisa

Busy! This is the one word that would describe my life during 2012. I had successfully raised two boys and was working on the third. I had obtained my bachelor's degree in English/teaching from Eastern Kentucky University and was in my fifth year of teaching drama at Lincoln County Middle School. I was just one semester away from earning my master's degree as a reading and writing specialist and was very busy taking a summer class toward this goal.

I was also enjoying my marriage to the fullest, going out with my husband and our close friends as often as time would allow. I was actively involved in my church, singing in the choir and helping with praise and worship when possible. Most of all, I was looking forward to the future. My husband and I were planning a cruise to celebrate our twenty-fifth anniversary.

Of course, things weren't all rosy. My middle son told me he was going

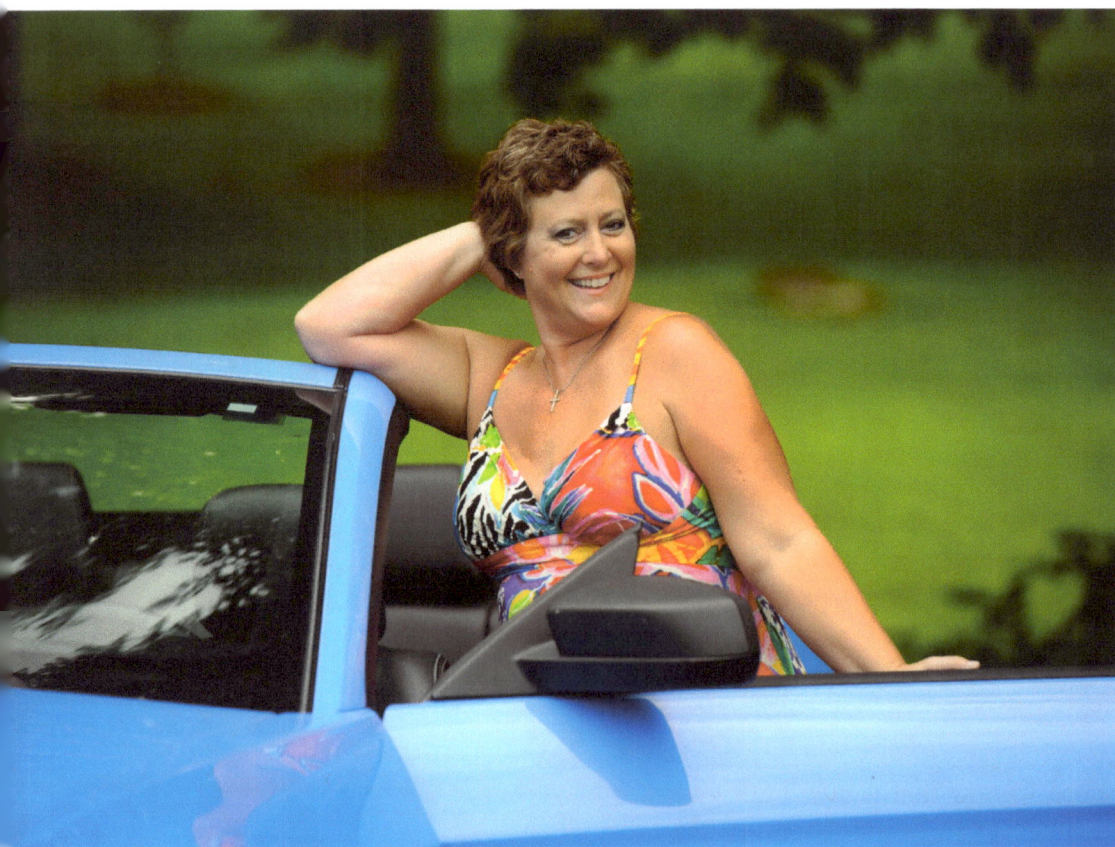

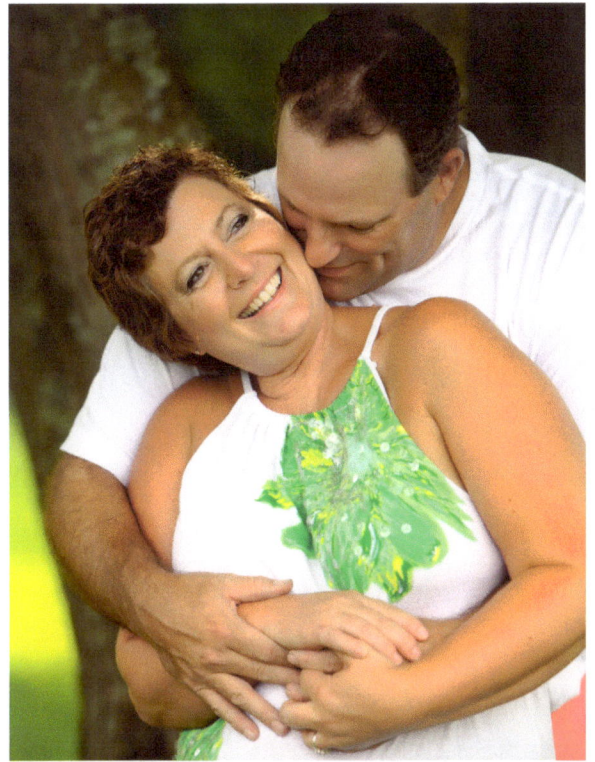

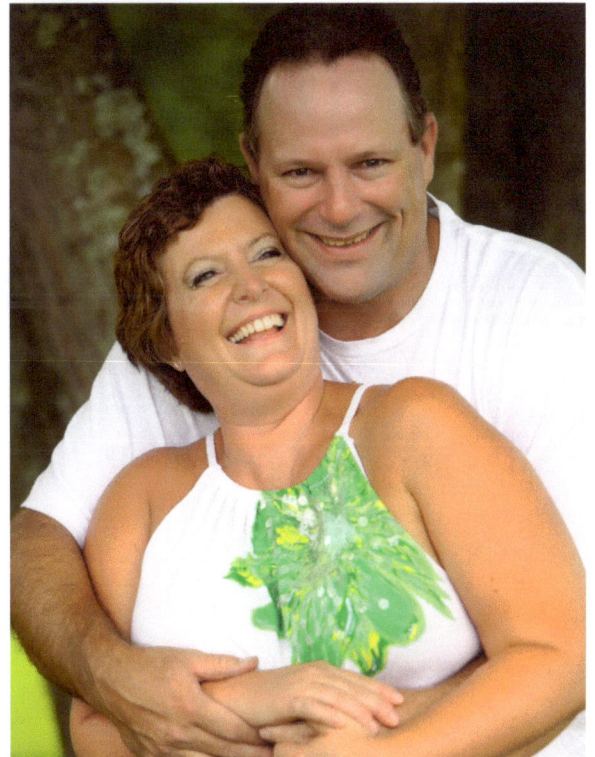

to the air force and would be called up to basic training at any time. I was very worried about this and knew that I would miss him, but he was making his own choices and growing up. That was a good thing. He left for air force basic training on June 19, 2012. It was a very difficult day for me—I spent the whole day in tears. My annual mammogram was scheduled for the following day, and I considered not going.

Previously, I'd had nothing but bad luck when it came to mammograms. I didn't think I could stand being called back in for more pictures, an ultrasound, or as usual, a biopsy of an abnormal spot. I was already so emotionally drained from Jarred leaving that I just wanted to stay home and not worry about anything else. But something told me not to cancel. I figured I would go, get it over with, and then head straight to class. I really needed to get an ultrasound done on a spot that had been biopsied six months before, so that my insurance would approve a breast reduction that I had wanted for so long.

During the mammogram, the technician told me that everything looked normal on both sides. I was relieved. I had just enough time to continue on with the ultrasound before I had to leave for class. And then, the ultrasound technician suddenly stopped to focus on one area. Looking at the monitor, I saw a star-shaped section that did not look like any of the spots I had ever had before. I knew that this was not good because it was not perfectly round and just looked different. The technician continued to measure and look without saying a word.

I'm really not sure why they do that. Most women are pretty smart and know when something is not right. Finally, the doctor came in and told me I needed a biopsy right away.

I explained that I had class and would need to schedule for another day. He sat me down in front of the computer and explained that with the size

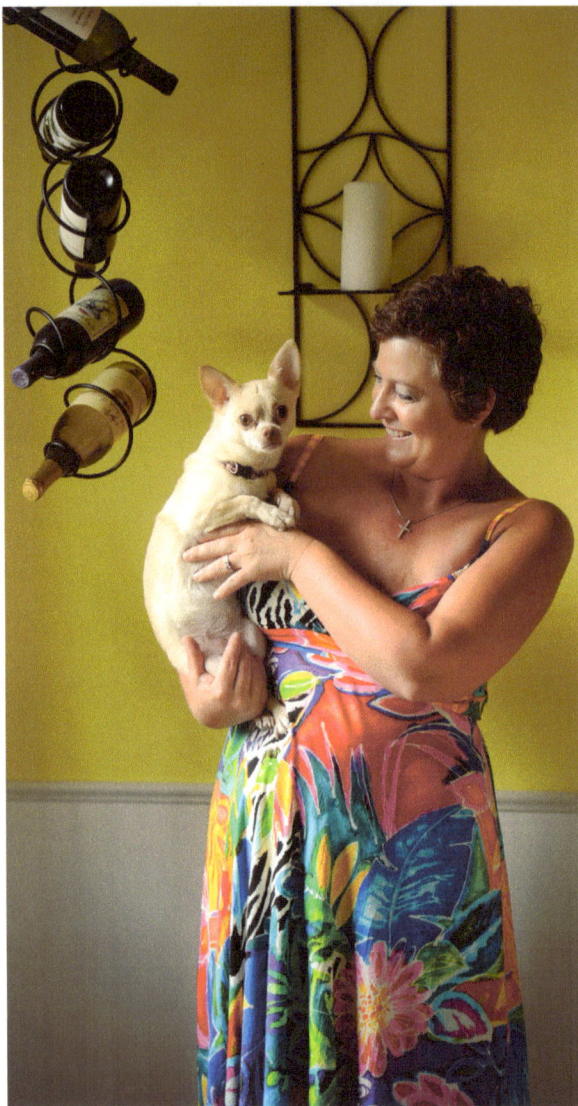

The next day I got the call that all women dread.

and shape of this spot, he was not comfortable letting me leave his office without the biopsy that very day. He was very serious as he told me that what he was seeing was very likely cancer, and we needed to get on it right away.

I had the biopsy (my fifth one in less than four years) and left that office with a bad feeling. Not only had my son just left for military basic training, but now my future was unknown, too. The next day I got the call that all women dread.

The you-have-breast-cancer call.

I was on my way to class. When the woman told me I might want to pull over, I told her just to tell me because I already knew. I remember feeling angry and so sick of my breasts because they'd caused me so many problems. "And now," I thought, "they're going to kill me!" Then, defiantly, "No, they are not!" My mantra suddenly became, Accept it, own it, kick its ass!

From the very first moment I knew I had breast cancer, I knew I wanted a double mastectomy. There was no doubt in my mind that I was ready for them both just to be taken off. I wanted to get into a surgeon as soon as possible. When I walked into my surgeon's office, he explained my options. He would take some lymph nodes to make sure the cancer had not spread, but in his opinion, a lumpectomy was all I needed.

I stopped him mid-speech and told him I wanted them both gone. No questions, just gone! Frankly, I was sick and tired of my breasts running my life.

He suggested I see a plastic surgeon before he operated. I turned him down flat. Something inside told me that my cancer, no matter how large, had not spread, and I wanted it off my body! My surgery was scheduled for July 5, 2012.

When I woke up, my surgeon said, "You have just been given Christmas in July. Your cancer was not in even one lymph node, and we got every last bit of it." I

"It is through my reconstruction that I feel like a woman again. A perfectly proportioned, alive, vivacious woman, who can achieve any goal I set my mind to."

was very relieved but still anxious to hear what my treatment would be.

I'll spare you the story of the anger, sadness, and depression that followed my surgery. I never really mourned the loss of my breasts, but I was scared to death about the prospect of chemo, and I missed my middle son with a passion. I questioned God about why he would take my son away and give me breast cancer—all in two very short days.

In August 2012, a week before my first chemotherapy treatment, I was able to attend Jarred's graduation into the United States Air Force Academy. It was one of the proudest moments of my life. He had made it through basic training, while I had made it through surgery and was headed toward the fight of my life.

When Jarred saw me for the first time that day, he was shocked. I hadn't told him about my diagnosis while he was still in training, and I'd been a 38 DD when he left home. Now, here I was—a nothing! After he got over the shock, he told me he'd thought I had my breast reduction, and they'd taken too much. We both got a good laugh out of that. He helped me so much that day by saying this: "Well, Mom, at least you're not going to die or anything."

I realized he was totally right. Life would go on. I would get through six chemo treatments and twelve months of Herceptin hormone therapy my oncologist had recommended. I would come out the other side a much stronger woman.

The treatments were not pleasant at all. There were times when I thought that I would not make it. Halfway into them, I started researching plastic surgeons. I knew now I wanted reconstructive surgery as soon as possible, but I did not know where to start. I had been so focused on getting the cancer off of my body that I'd given very little thought to the reconstructive process. I narrowed my search down to a couple of plastic surgeons in the Lexington area

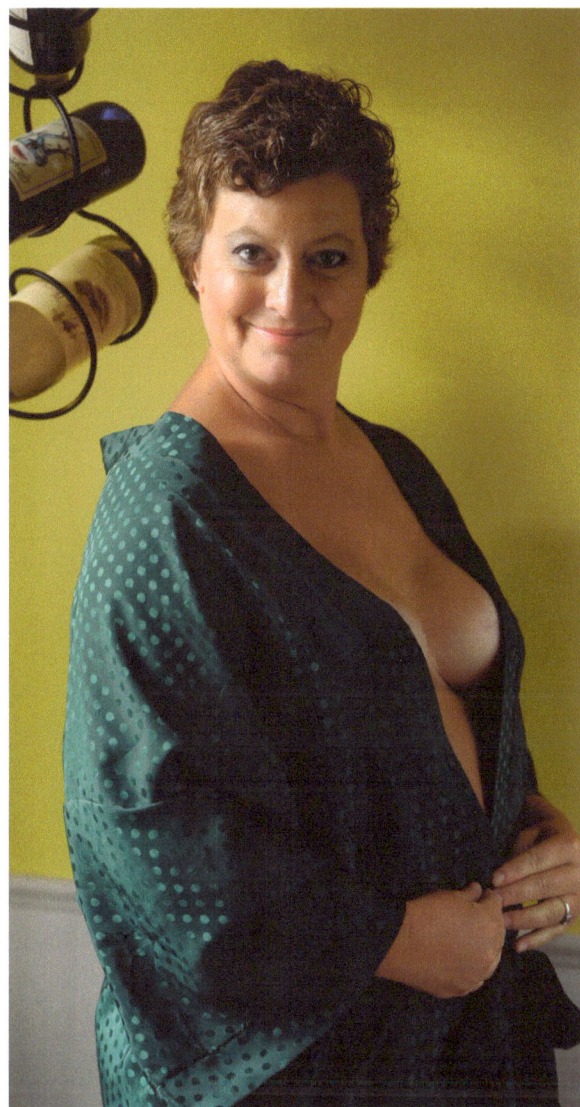

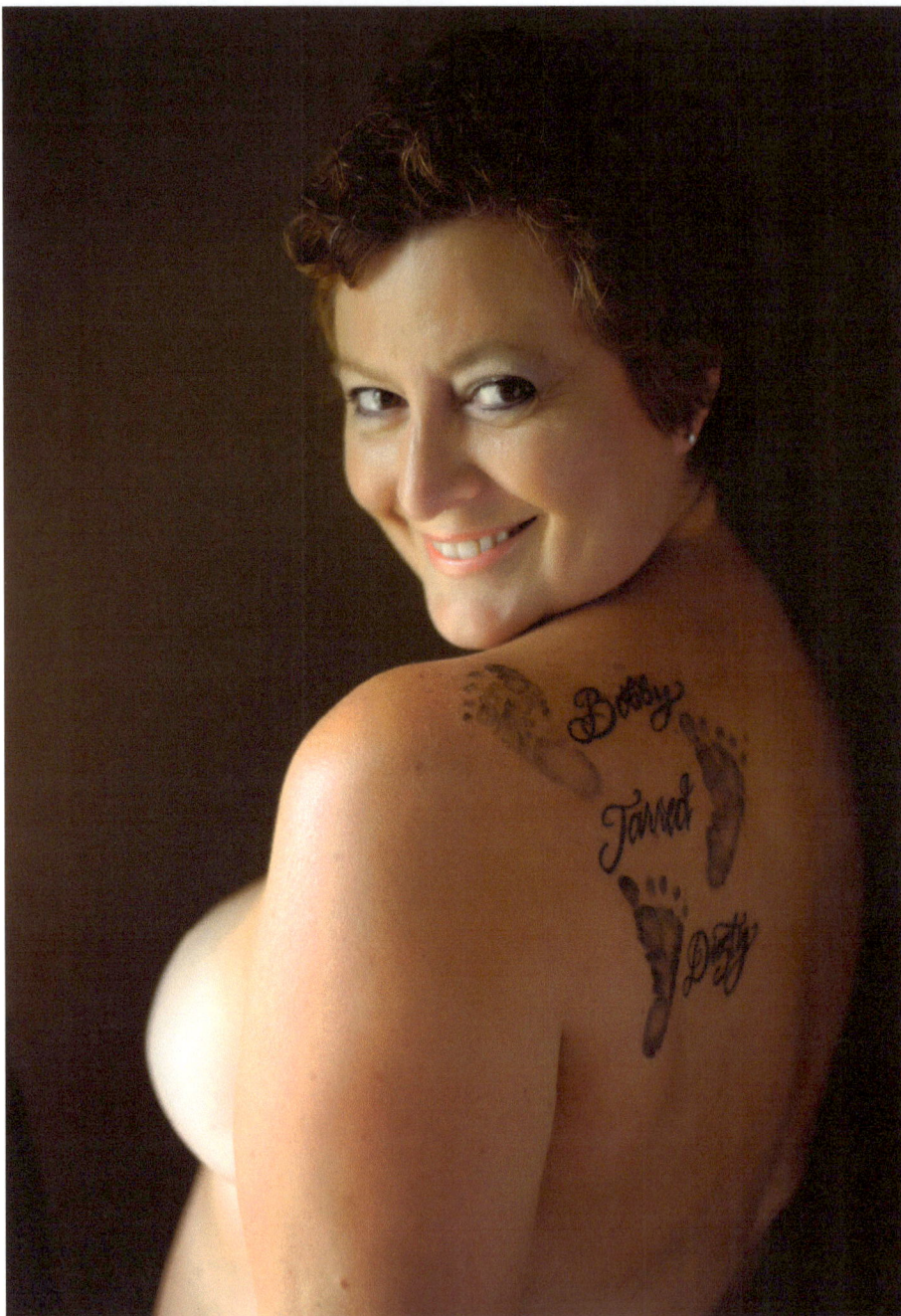

and finally decided on Dr. Bouzaglou.

I had heard several friends rave about her during support groups at the Lexington Clinic and had also seen her work firsthand. (If you are not aware, women who have had reconstruction after breast cancer love to show off their new "girls.") I knew that my case was going to be a little more of a challenge because I'd had the traditional sideways incisions. I wanted a talented plastic surgeon who loved a good challenge.

My life and my perspective on breast cancer surgery totally changed when I walked into the plastic surgery center on October 4. Feeling very sad, I explained that it was my fault I had not seen her before my mastectomy. I had just wanted them gone, even though my surgeon tried to get me to have a plastic surgeon mark my incisions. But this doctor was excited about all the extra skin that my surgeon had left her. She assured me that I was still a good candidate for expanders and permanent implants, once my chemo was complete.

I don't want to dwell on how awful the next few months were, but I will say this: I would not wish breast cancer treatments on my worst enemy. At the same time, I know that those treatments saved my life. They reduced my chance of ever get-

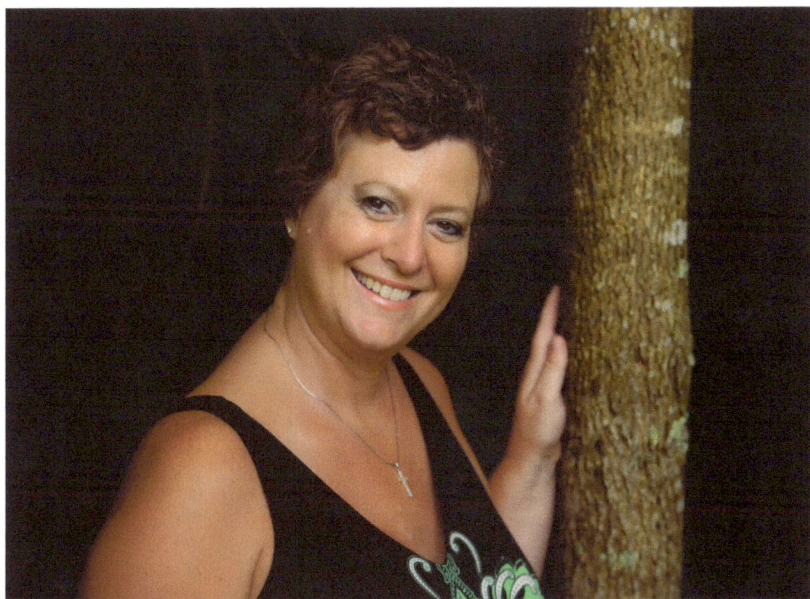

ting breast cancer again to less than 13 percent. I will be forever grateful to my doctors and caregivers. They gave me the best care possible.

I will also always be thankful that I found Dr. Bouzaglou and her wonderful staff. It is through my reconstruction that I feel like a woman again. A perfectly proportioned, alive, vivacious woman, who can achieve any goal I set my mind to.

My goal here is to make every woman not only aware of how important early detection is but also how important it is to have a plastic surgeon involved from the very first mastectomy or lumpectomy consultation. I have been blessed with wonderful results, but that is rare with the type of incision I had.

I want women to know that there is life after your diagnosis and after surgery. Eventually, you are going to want to feel like a woman again, beautiful breasts and all. Please take the time to consider a plastic surgeon before your initial procedure for breast cancer.

If I've learned anything though this experience, it is that, with faith in God and support from a wonderful family, it's possible to get through any hardship and come out on the other side a much better person than before.

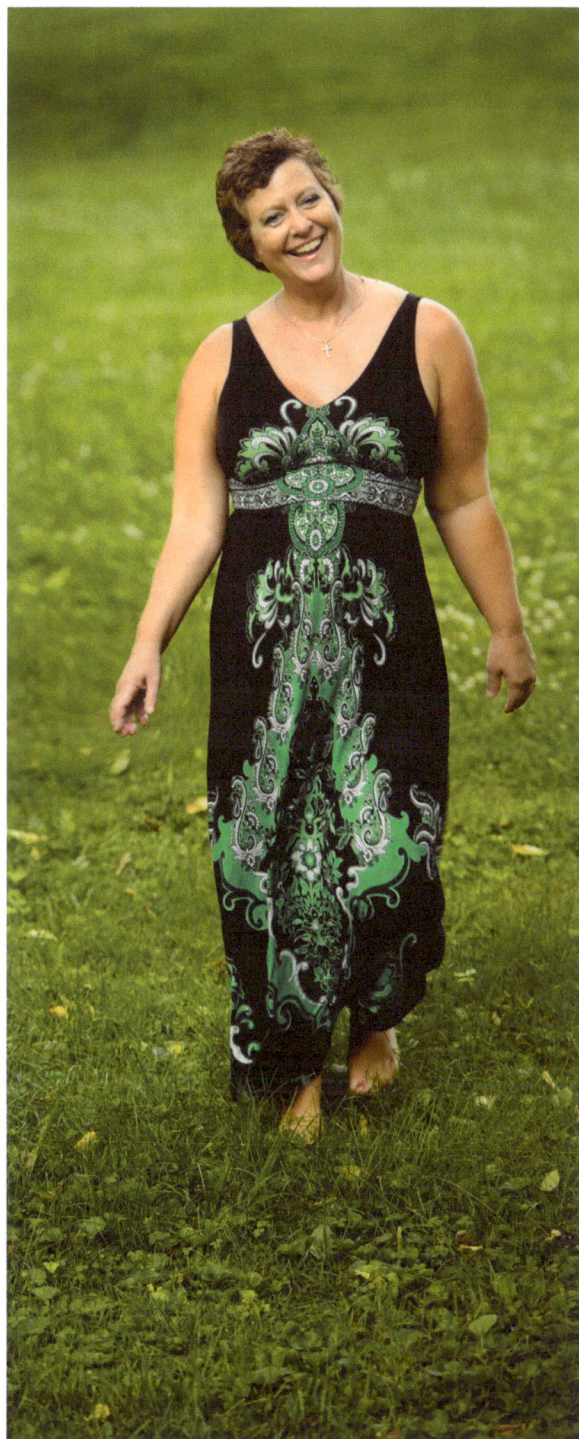

Shawna

I am a wife, a mother of three, a two-time breast cancer survivor, and this is my story.

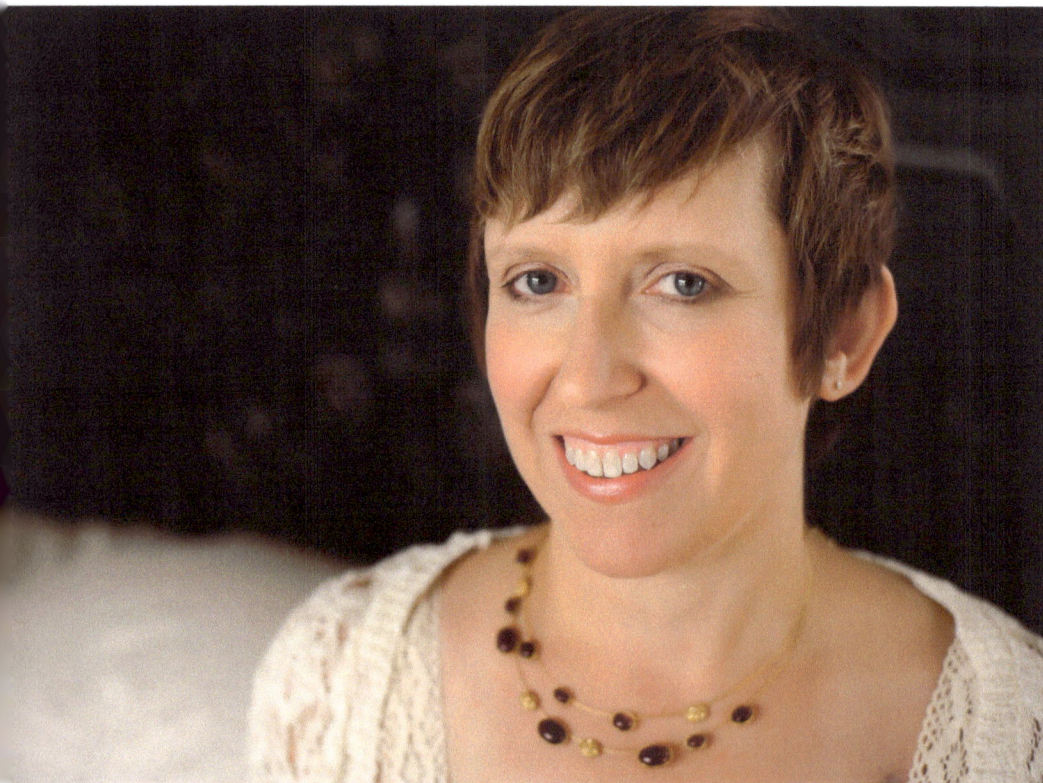

In December 2008, during a routine baseline mammogram at the age of forty, some calcifications were spotted on my right breast. I was given the choice of waiting six months to repeat the mammogram or do a biopsy. I chose the biopsy.

The calcifications turned out to be DCIS breast cancer. I chose the most conservative treatment: a lumpectomy and five days of radiation per week for seven weeks. I had my lumpectomy on New Year's Eve 2008. The tumor turned out to be triple negative, so no further treatment was given.

In January 2012, calcifications were once again discovered on my right breast during a routine mammogram. Given my history, a biopsy was scheduled immediately. This time, the diagnosis was a small invasive breast cancer.

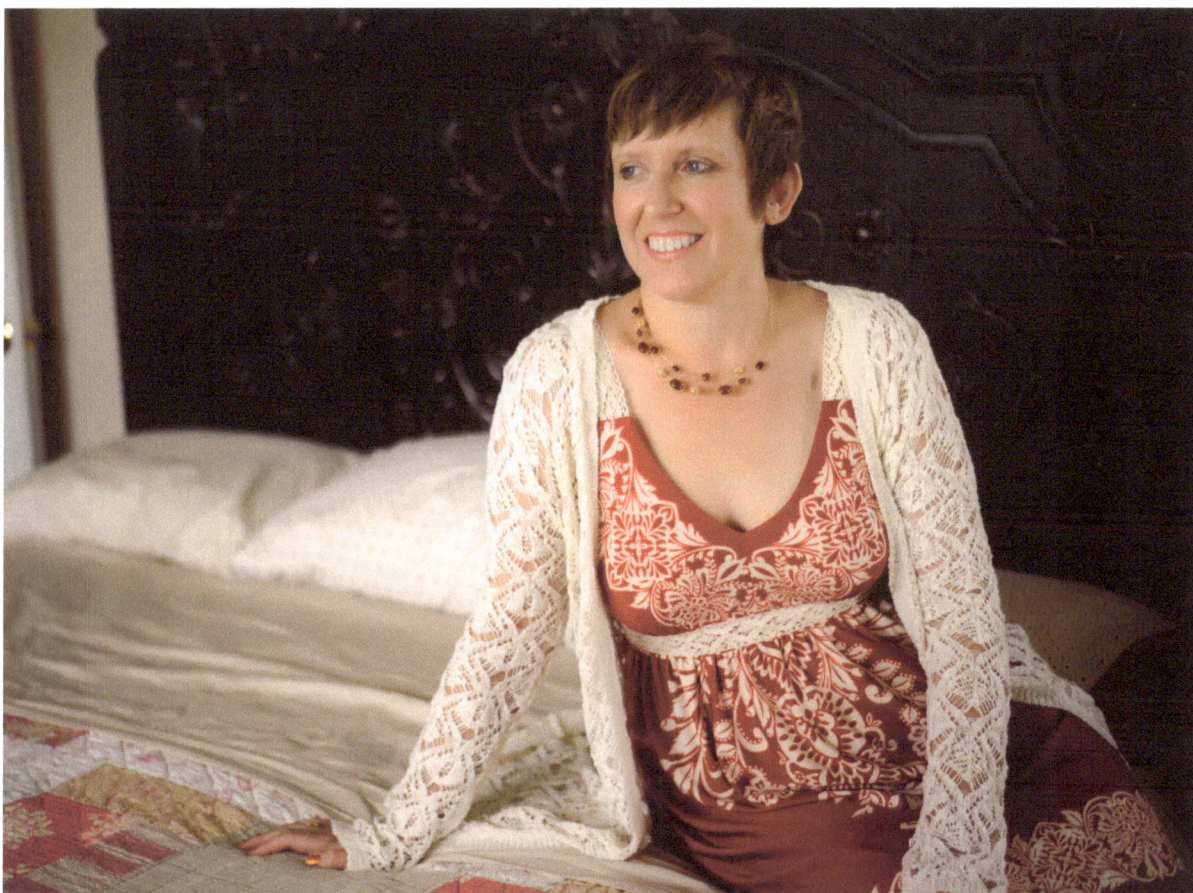

I elected a bilateral mastectomy rather than a life of living mammogram to mammogram. After some online research, I knew I wanted reconstructive surgery. I learned that the best results are achieved when a plastic surgeon is involved during the mastectomy. Before surgery, I interviewed a couple of plastic surgeons to find the best fit for me but my case was not an easy one.

Since I'd had radiation in the past, most plastic surgeons did not want to do implants on radiated tissue. I was told that I did not have enough belly fat to do a flap for two breasts. I could do one breast that way and an implant for the other breast. That just sounded too complicated. I chose to try an implant for both breasts.

The plastic surgeon I chose to work with met with me the day before my mastectomy to design the incisions for the surgeon to follow. During the surgery, tissue expanders were put into place. This time, my small, invasive tumor turned out to be triple positive,

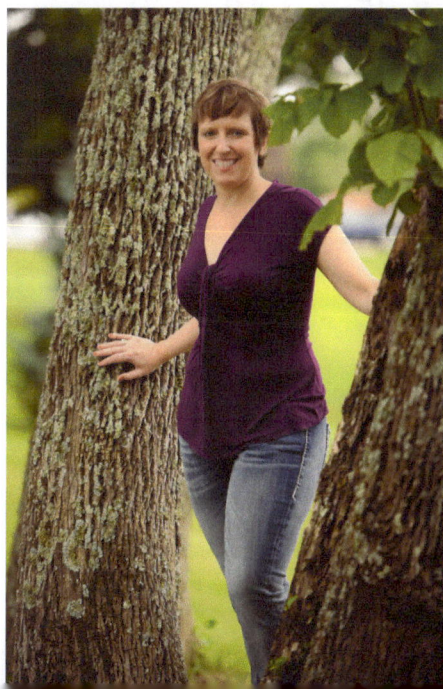

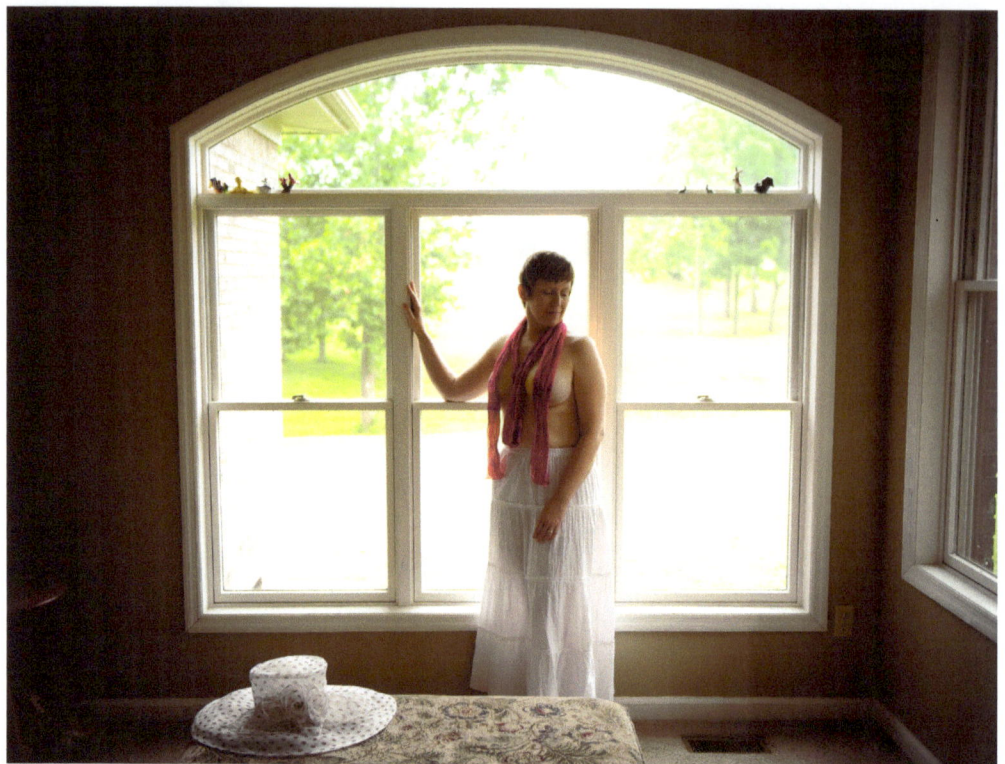

"My surgeon has worked her magic and I think I look even better than before the reconstructive surgery."

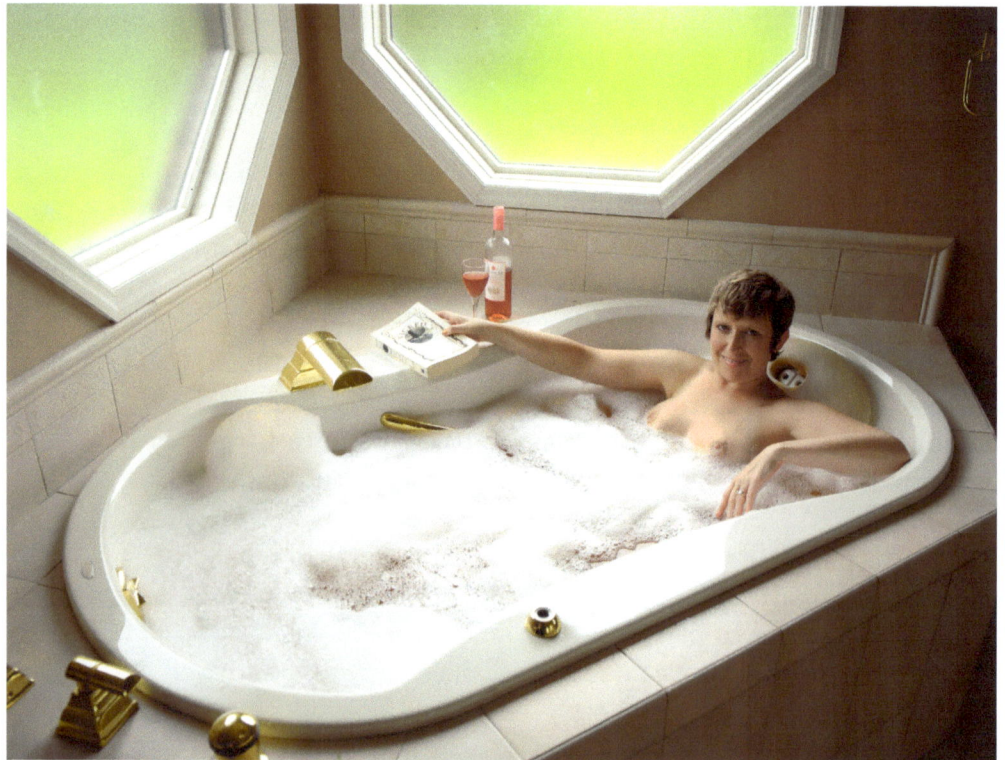

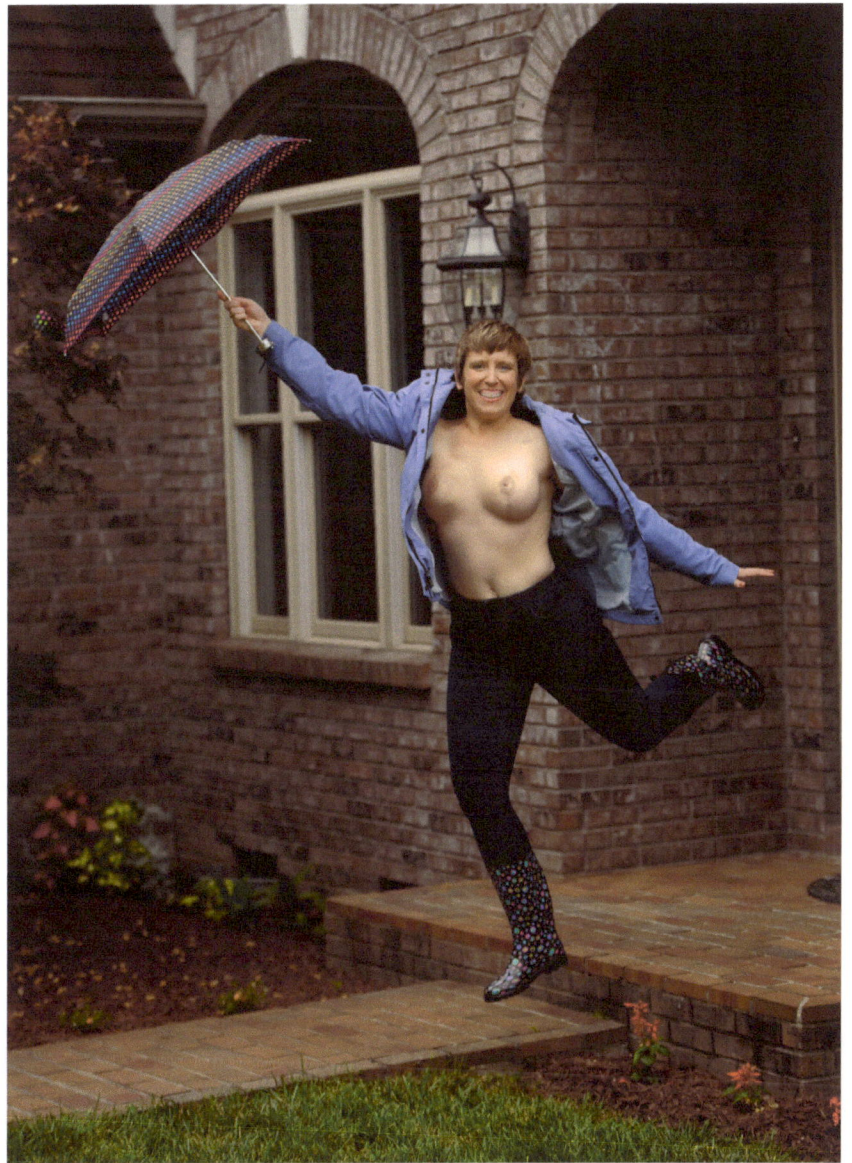

which meant six rounds of chemotherapy and a year of Herceptin. I put my reconstructive surgery on hold while I completed the chemotherapy.

Going to Dr. Bouzaglou was a lot more fun than going to the oncologist. The oncologist was always telling me how bad the chemotherapy was going to make me feel, and that my hair was going to fall out. Dr. B kept telling me how well I was doing, and how great I was going to look. That helped a lot, especially on the days I didn't feel so good. Finally, I finished my chemotherapy and could complete my reconstructive surgery.

I had my expanders replaced with implants in September 2012. The left side had not had radiation in the past and looked great. The right side was a little more difficult. The first implant was higher and firmer than the one on the left. It also started to feel painful.

Dr. Bouzaglou wanted to try again. She replaced the right implant in April 2013. This time, I tried massaging the implant. The massaging put stress on the incision and caused it to gape open in places but after a scary episode, the incision healed. The massage worked and the right breast looks better than I could have ever hoped.

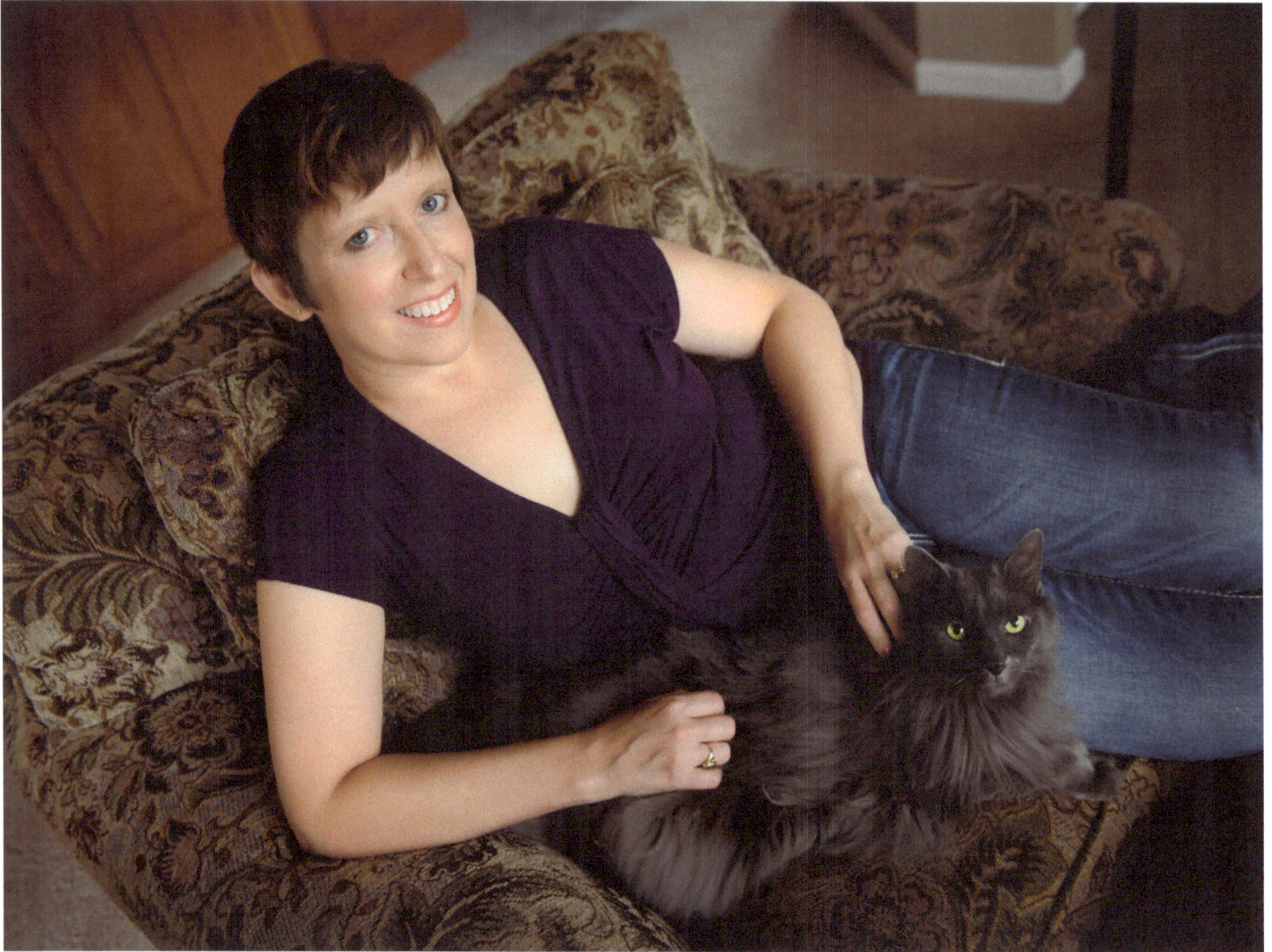

I still have a couple of procedures left to complete my reconstructive surgery, but I am so thrilled with my results. My surgeon has worked her magic and I think I look even better than before the reconstructive surgery. If I had known how great reconstructive surgery results could be, I would have chosen the bilateral mastectomy at the time of my first diagnosis.

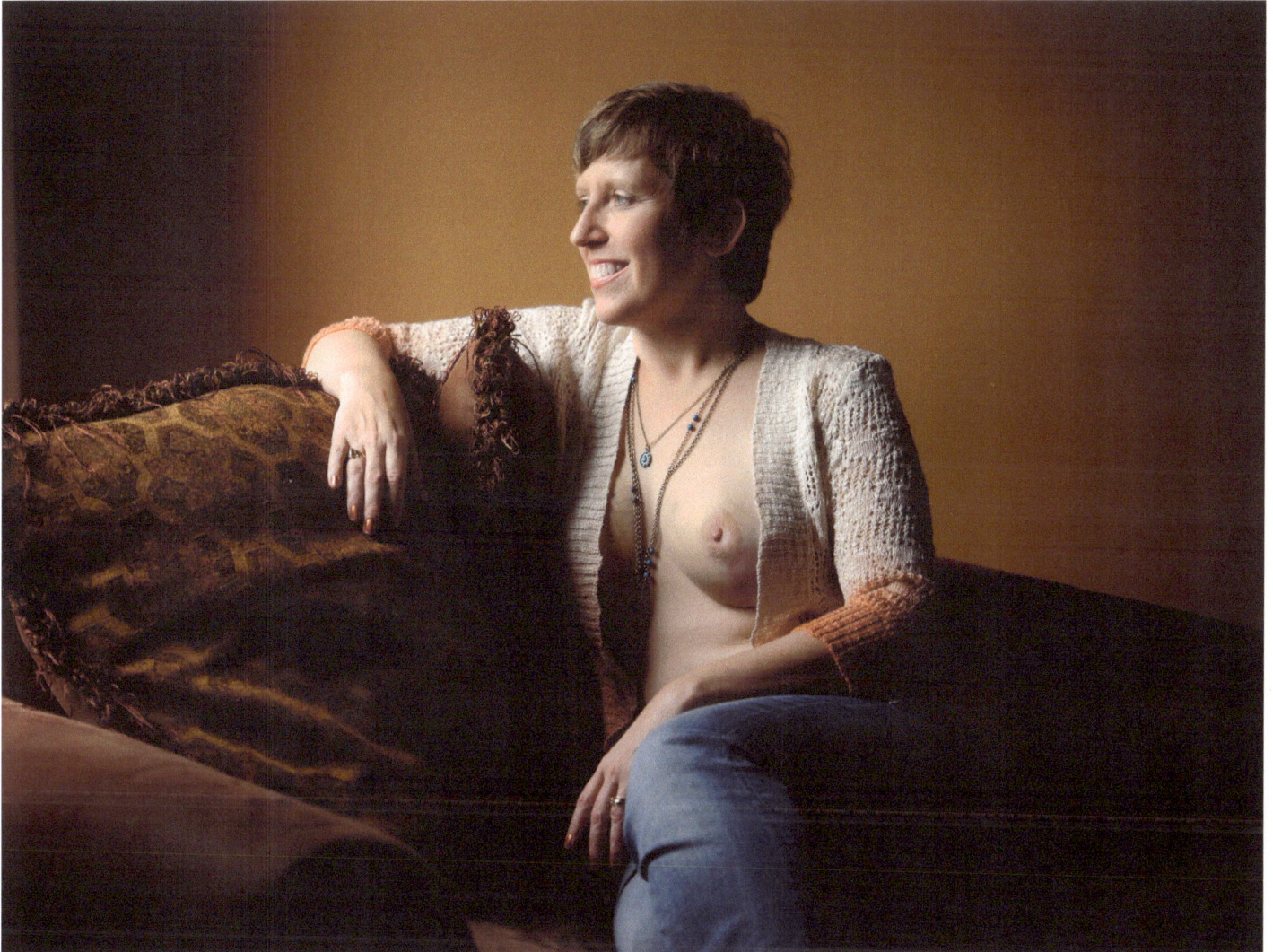

It's a wonderful thing to look in the mirror and feel like yourself after the difficult journey of breast cancer treatment. I feel so blessed to have found my plastic surgeon. She made me whole again after a terrible disease threatened to take that away.

Marsha

It was Valentine's Day, 2003.

I had started lifting weights, and for a few days I felt a pain in my right breast. I thought it was a muscle, but started rubbing and felt a lump! It felt like a grape inside my breast. It wasn't rock hard, and it was moveable.

Being a world-class hypochondriac with a gold medal in jumping to conclusions, I realized that I had breast cancer and was going to die.

The next Monday, I called my OBGYN and reported that I had a lump. They made an appointment for the following Monday. Then, the Great Ice Storm of 2003 happened. Fortunately, my OBGYN's office opened by Monday and I scampered in.

"Remember, cancer doesn't hurt," said the nurse, unhelpfully.

I smiled sadly at her.

OBGYN came in and felt my breast. I saw a brief "Oh, shit,"

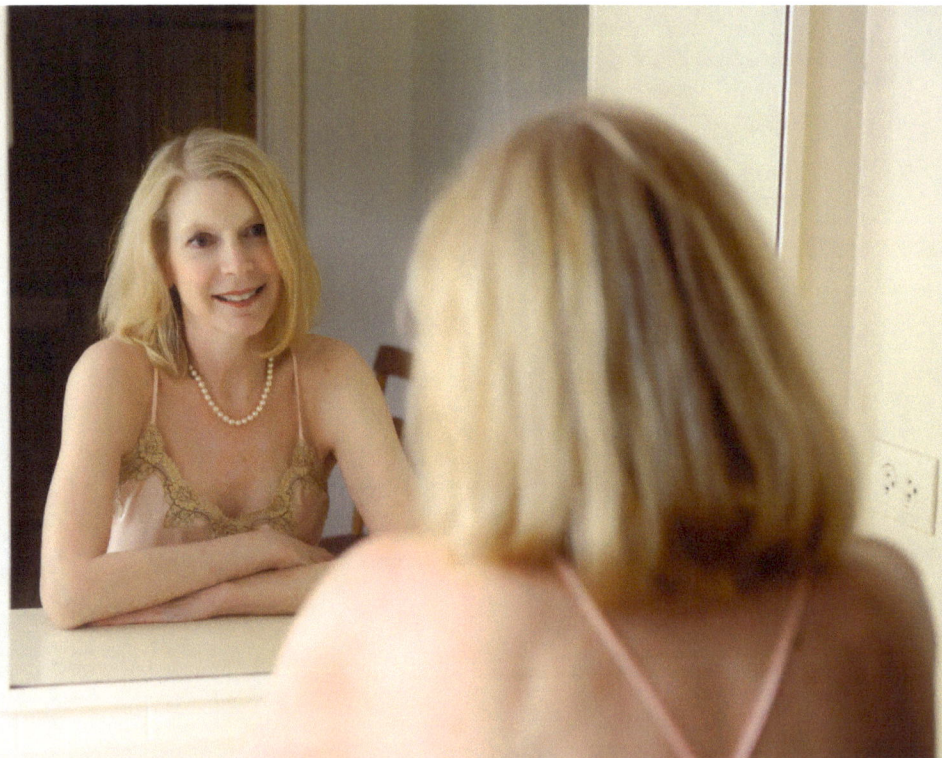

look cross his face.

"It's probably a fibroadenoma," he said, "but I'd like you to have a mammogram TOMORROW." Then, he hastened to the phone to set up the mammogram.

Tuesday, I went to the mammogram place, where everyone repeated the "Oh, shit," look and compared my mammogram from ten months ago.

"It was clean as a whistle last April," said the tech.

They asked me to come in for a biopsy TOMORROW. Wednesday, I went for the biopsy.

The doctor doing the biopsy said, "It's worrisome for a cancer." She shot the biopsy gun into my breast several times.

I remember looking at a pretty picture of flowers on the wall in the room and thinking, "This is it. This is the way the world ends. I'm gonna die."

The doctor then called the expert breast surgeon, and he wanted to see me TOMORROW. Thursday, I went into see the expert breast surgeon. He felt my poor boob, which was swollen after the biopsy.

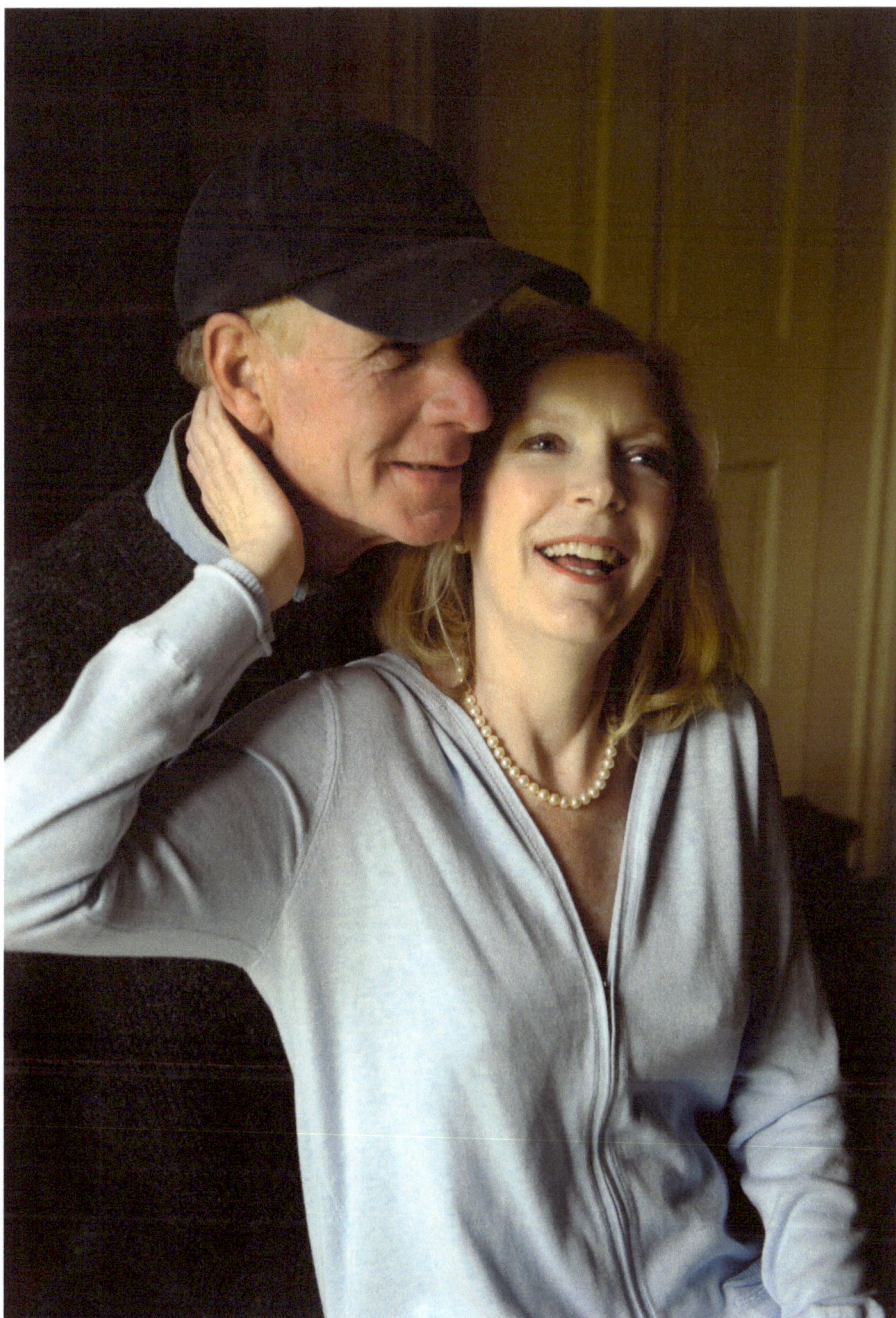

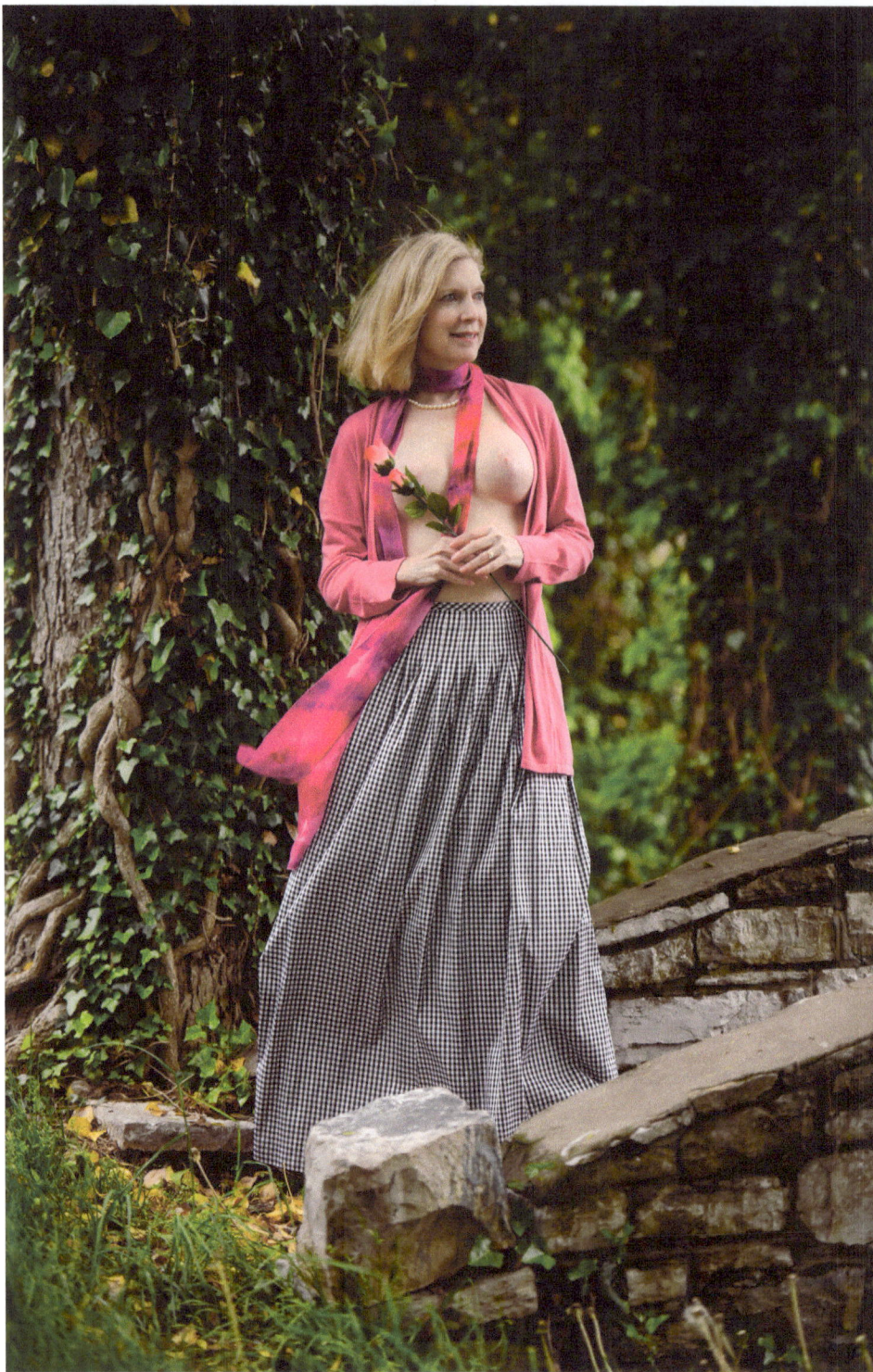

He said, "I am leaving for an exclusive breast surgeon convention but I can do your mastectomy or lumpectomy TOMORROW."

Then, he went into the whole song and dance about mastectomy vs. lumpectomy and radiation and if I did the mastectomy, I could get the reconstruction later.

The biopsy doctor bursts into the room. "It's better than we thought," he said. "Her tumor is only Grade 2, not Grade 3."

The expert breast surgeon, who had been as grave as an undertaker during the whole proceeding, looked somewhat cheered.

I said, "Let's just do the mastectomy."

Nobody mentioned a plastic surgeon at that point and since everything seemed to need to done immediately, I never thought that one could be rounded up by the next day.

The next day, I had the mastectomy. "The tumor was smaller than we

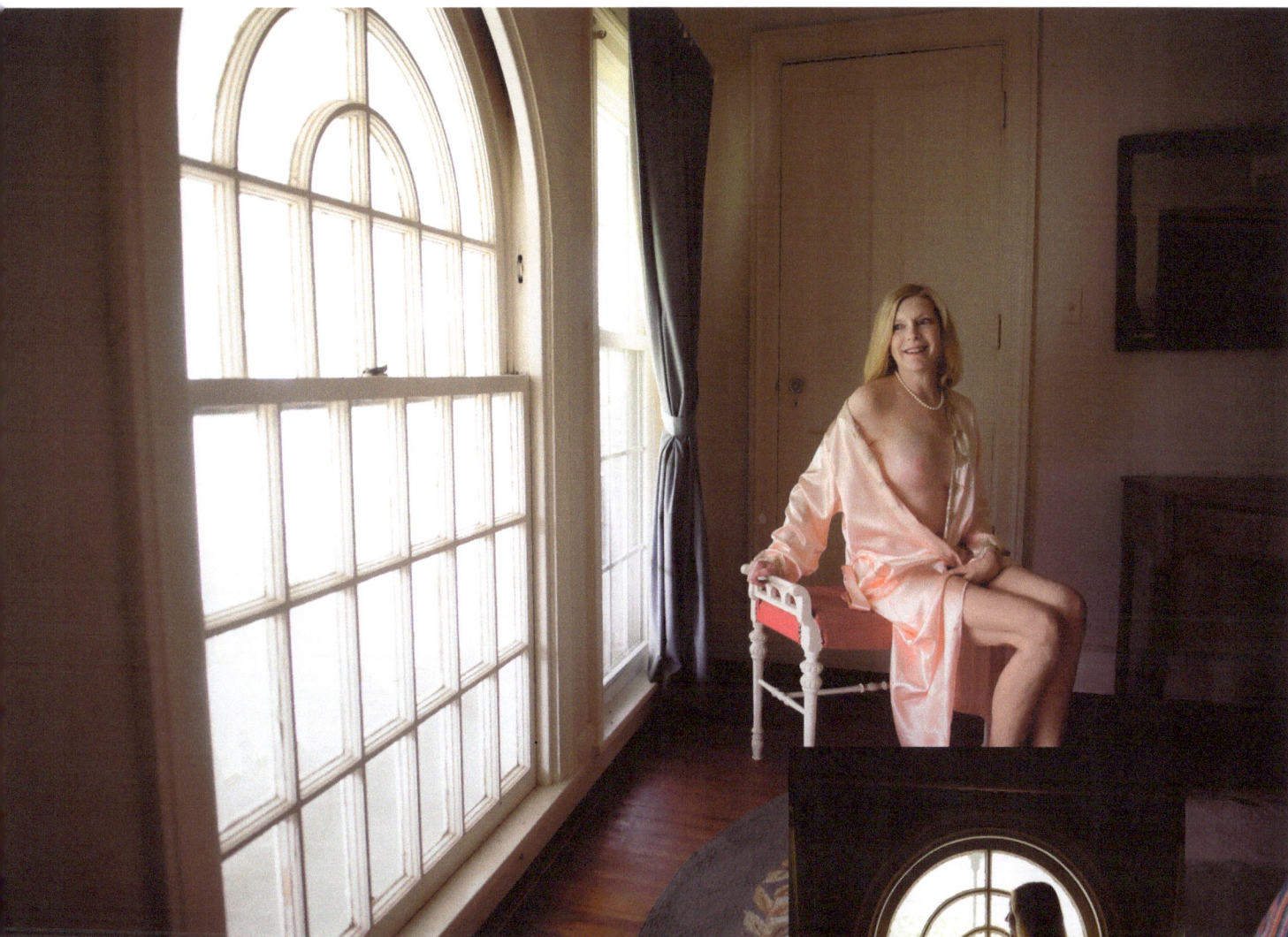

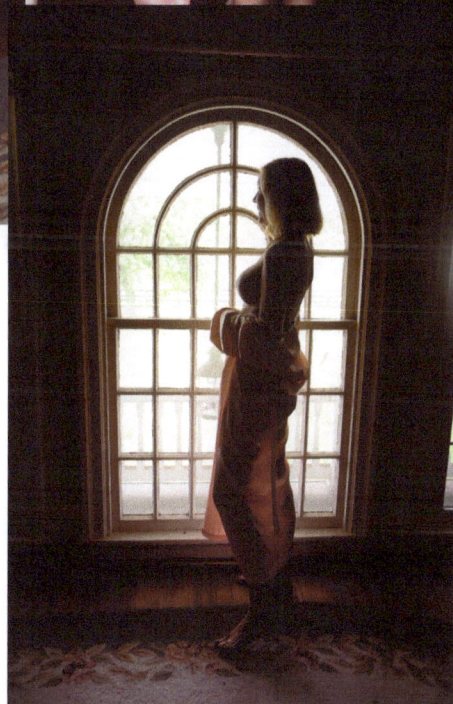

thought," the breast surgeon informed me.

The mastectomy didn't really hurt and there weren't complications, but I could tell the uniboob look was not for me.

Since I was the dreaded Triple Negative, with a poor prognosis, I started chemo. After chemo, I did research on reconstruction. My oncologist in Danville recommended a plastic surgeon, and I made an appointment. I knew that I insurance would pay for a prophylactic mastectomy on the other side and reconstruction, and that is what we decided to do.

It wasn't fun, but it was something to do while my hair grew back, and the results have been great.

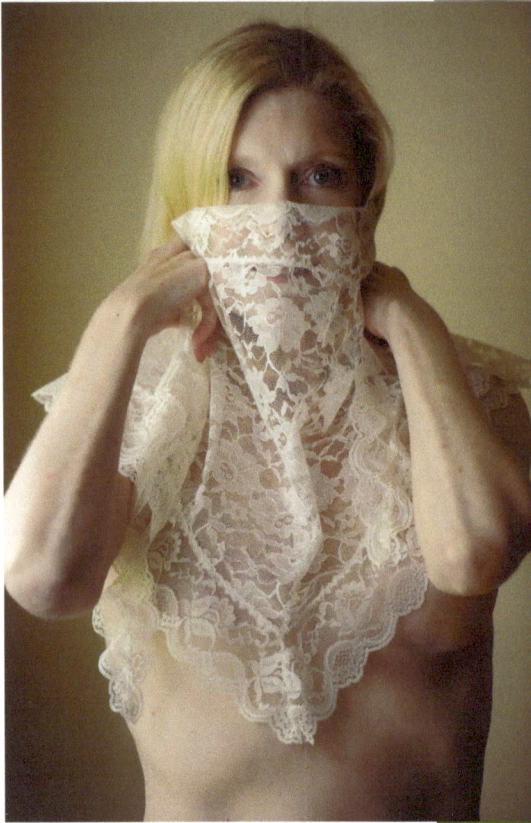

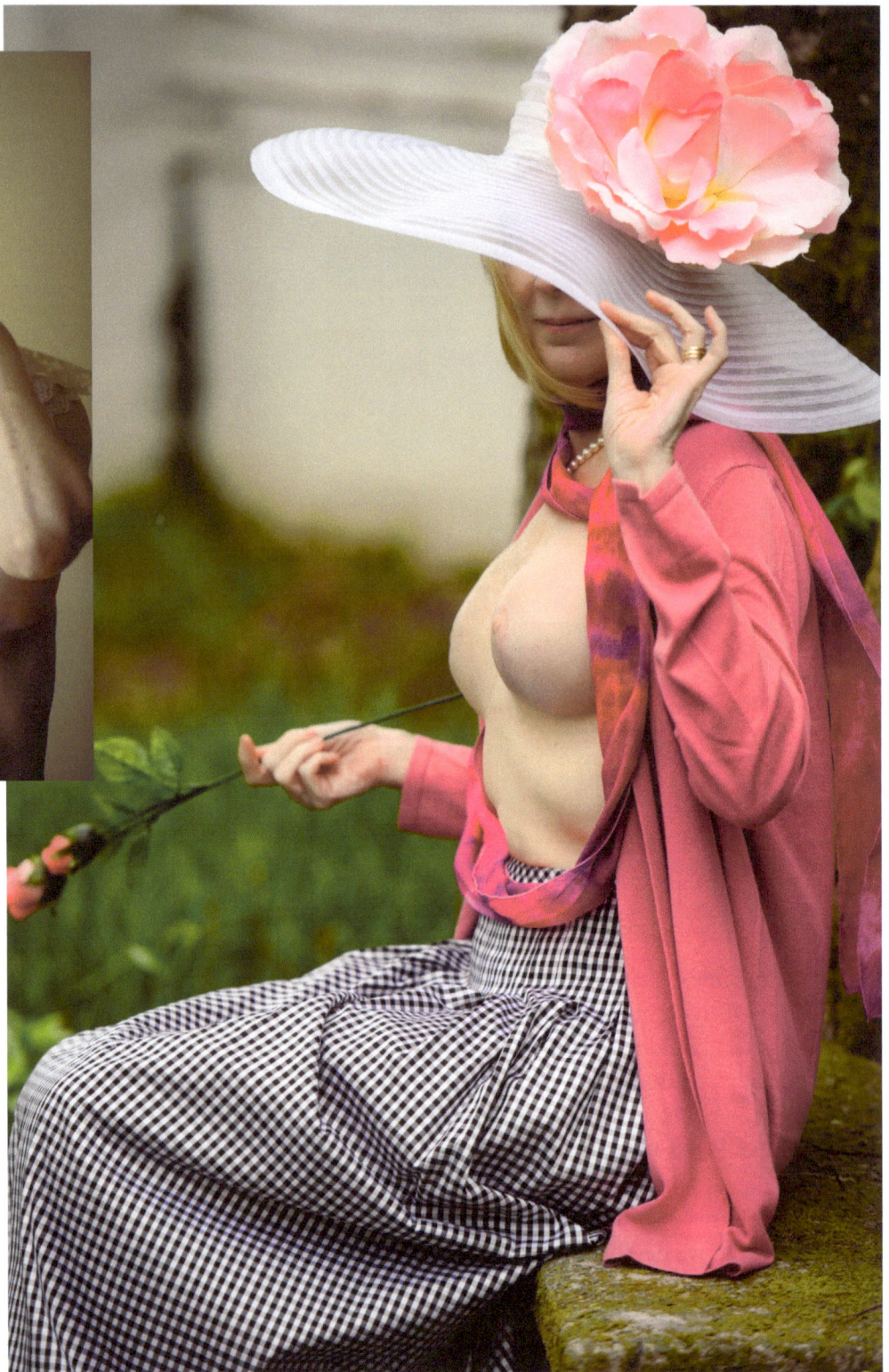

"*Reconstruction was just as important to my psychological well being as chemo was to my physical well-being. I look better than I did before cancer!*"

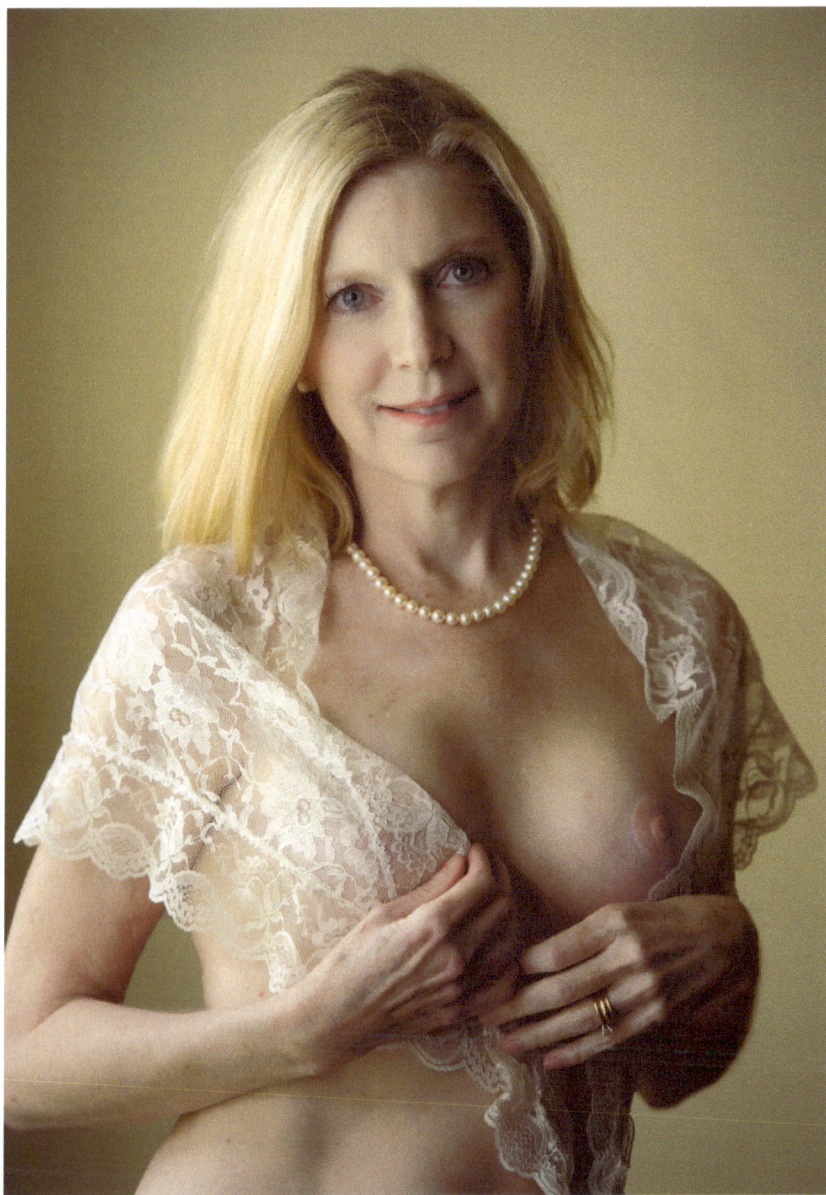

Reconstruction was the first thing that made me feel like I wasn't going to die, and that I was still a person, not just a cancer patient.

Reconstruction was just as important to my psychological well being as chemo was to my physical well-being. I look better than I did before cancer!

And P.S. I did not die.

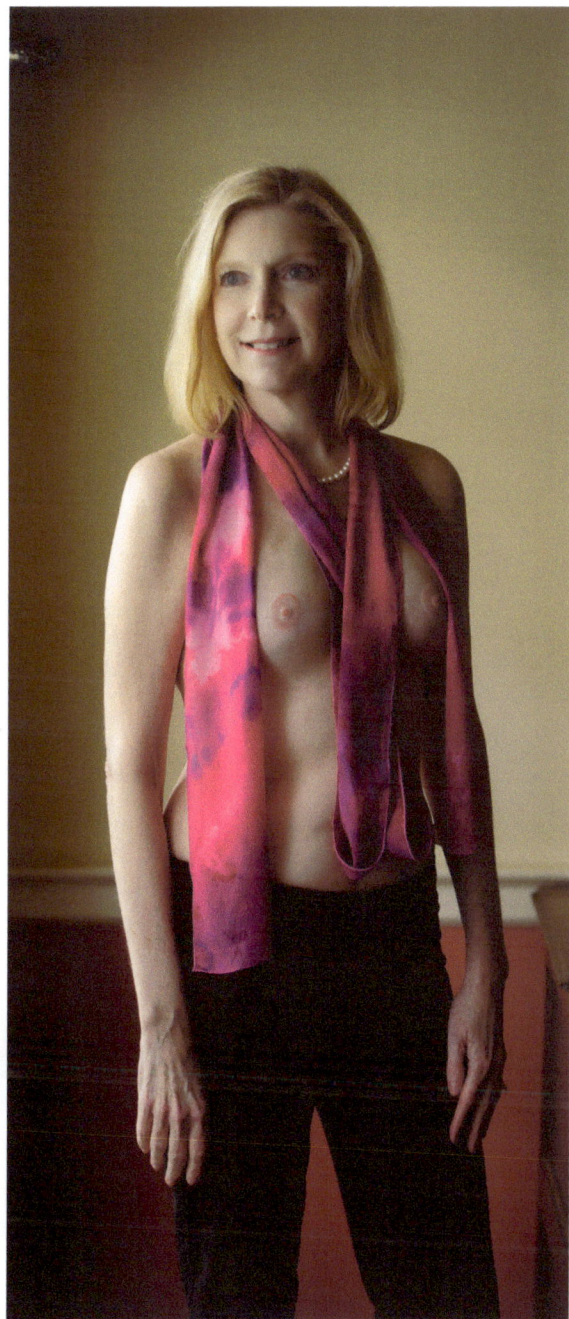

Holly

In February of 2009 after a miscarriage, I thought I might be pregnant again.

At this time, I had five-year old and three-year old little girls. My three-year old jumped on my lap in the recliner so I could read her a book. When she sat back on me I could feel soreness in my left breast. When I got to feeling around, I felt a small lump.

The next day, I found out I was pregnant.

After miscarrying, I waited until I was about eight weeks pregnant again before going to my OB. I mentioned the lump to my doctor who thought it was probably just a Fibro Adenoma. She decided to have it

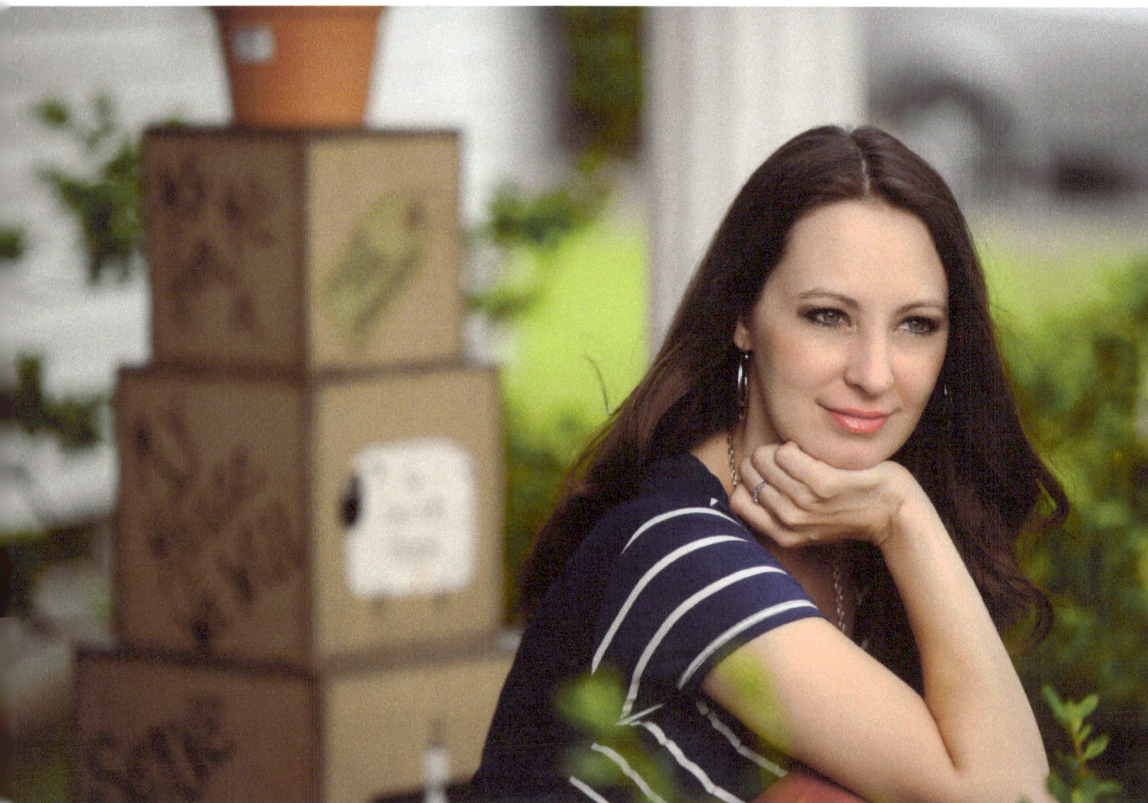

ultra sounded just to be safe.

The office called about four days later. They recommended I see a general surgeon but he didn't think it was anything to worry about, either. He wanted to schedule a biopsy but my whole family ended up catching the flu.

Another three weeks passed before I could even have the biopsy. By then, the place had gotten bigger, so we decided to do a lumpectomy to remove what was most likely a cyst.

On April 20, 2009, I had a lumpectomy performed with only local numbing meds.

On April 21, 2009, at seventeen weeks pregnant, the general surgeon told me that I had breast cancer.

I was in SHOCK! Breast cancer didn't run in my family and I had followed all the rules!

I asked the doctor for my options. The first thing he told me was to terminate my pregnancy and continue as a cancer patient. Quickly, I told him that was NOT an option.

I was ready to fight this! Nothing was taking me away from my babies! I knew with God on my side and a good attitude I could do this!

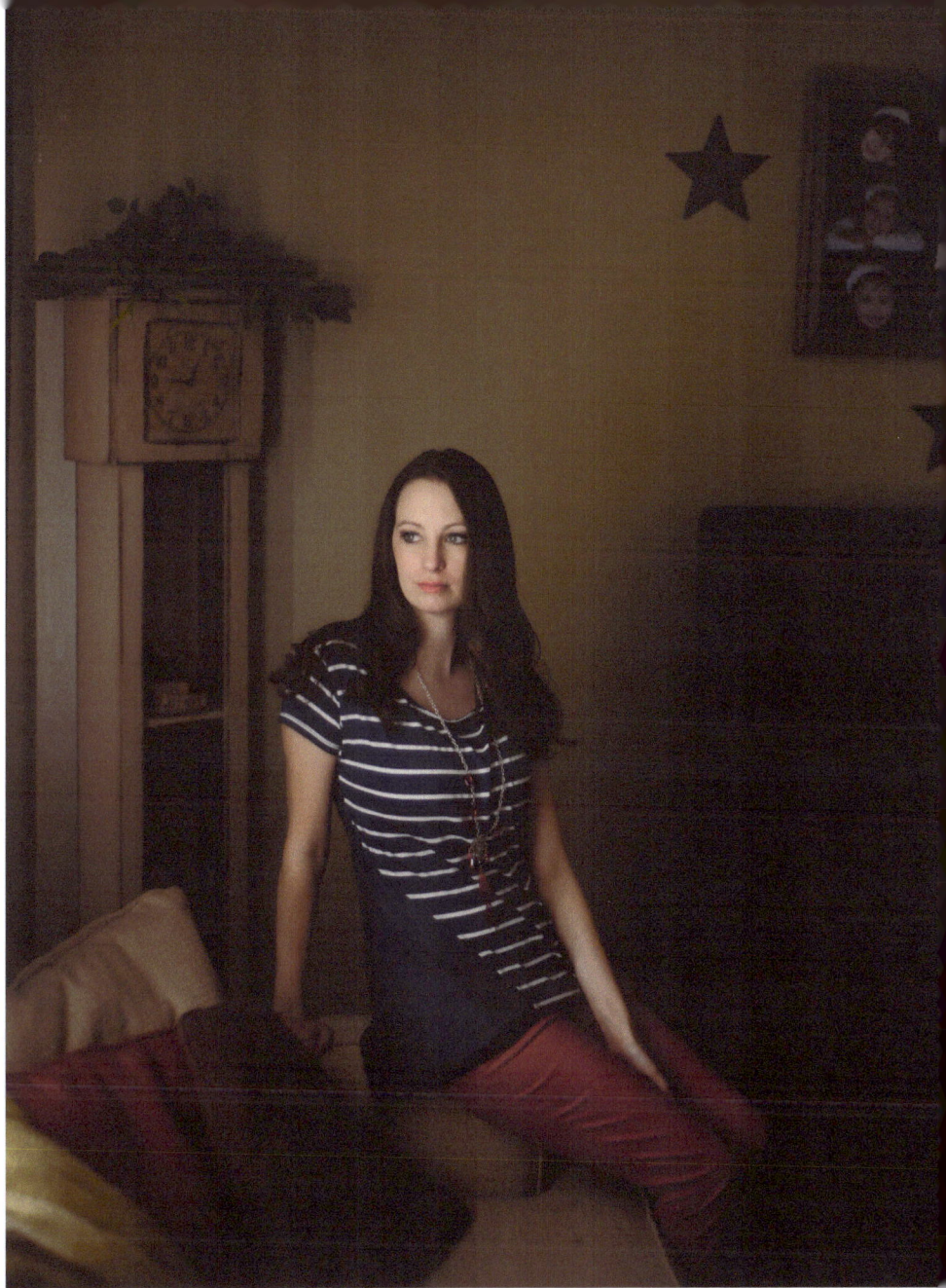

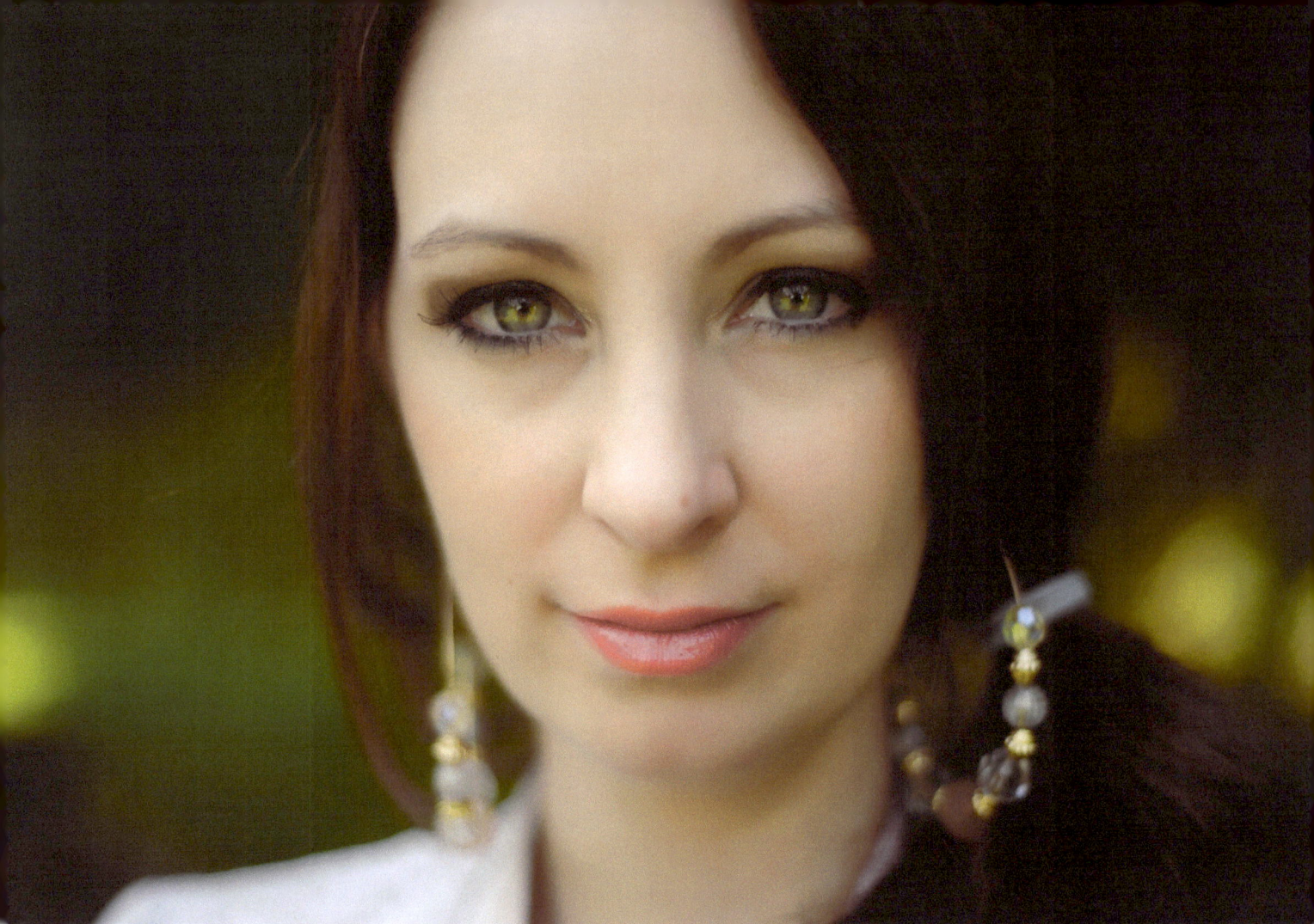

"I can't even express the feeling of having MY breasts back. I feel like a woman again!"

I went home and started searching for a good oncologist. Every office I called was negative and gave me excuses about how being pregnant would make the cancer hard to work with. Finally, after calling about ten different places, I talked to a lady that was so positive and uplifting; I knew that's where I needed to be.

I made an appointment and met all the doctors. They told me I was at a perfect time (twenty weeks) in my pregnancy to have a mastectomy and I could even do the chemo I would need while pregnant! When I was thirty-two weeks, they would induce me so that I could start another type of chemo that wasn't as safe for the baby.

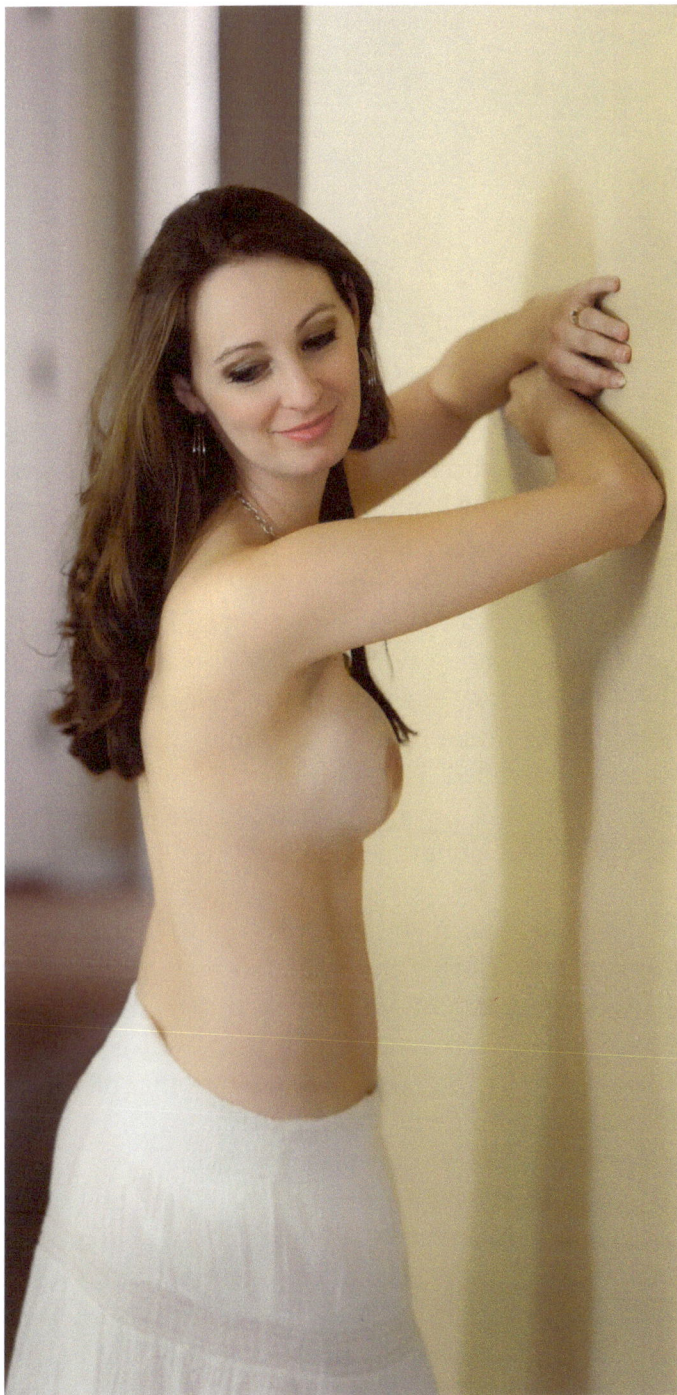

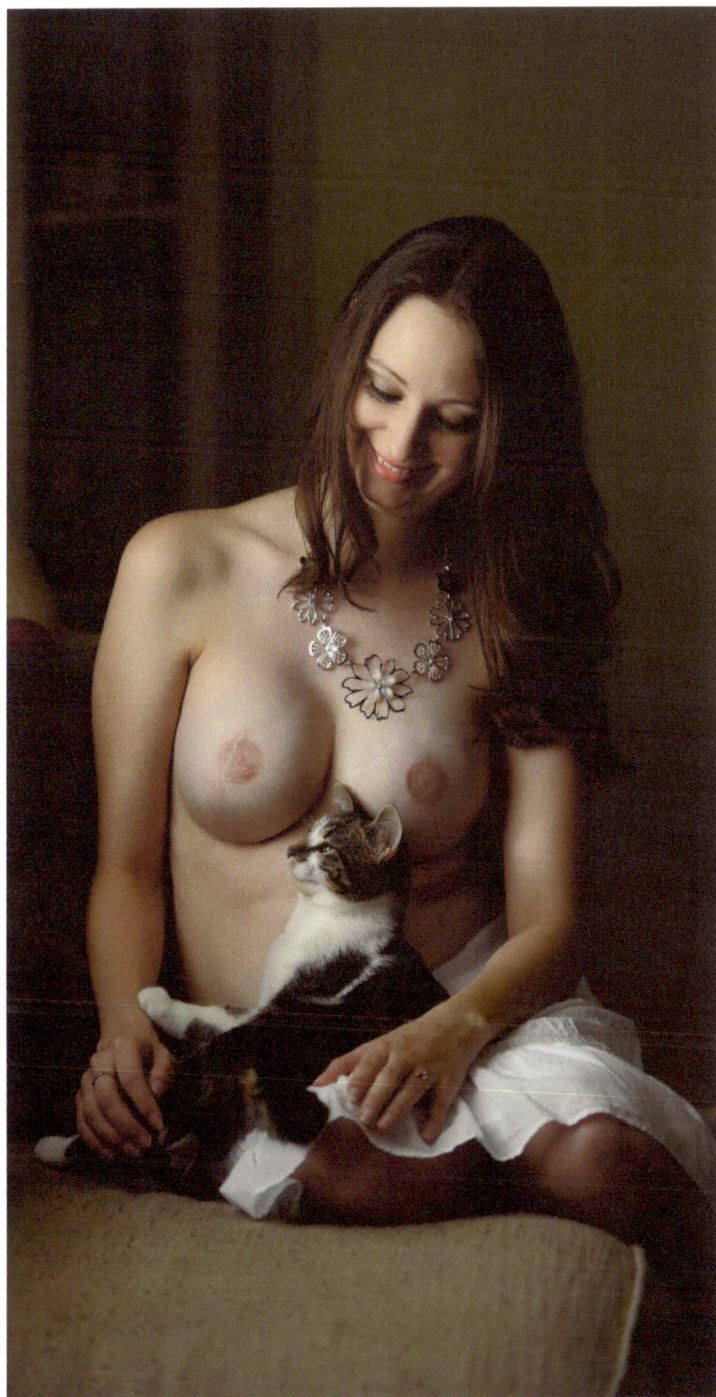

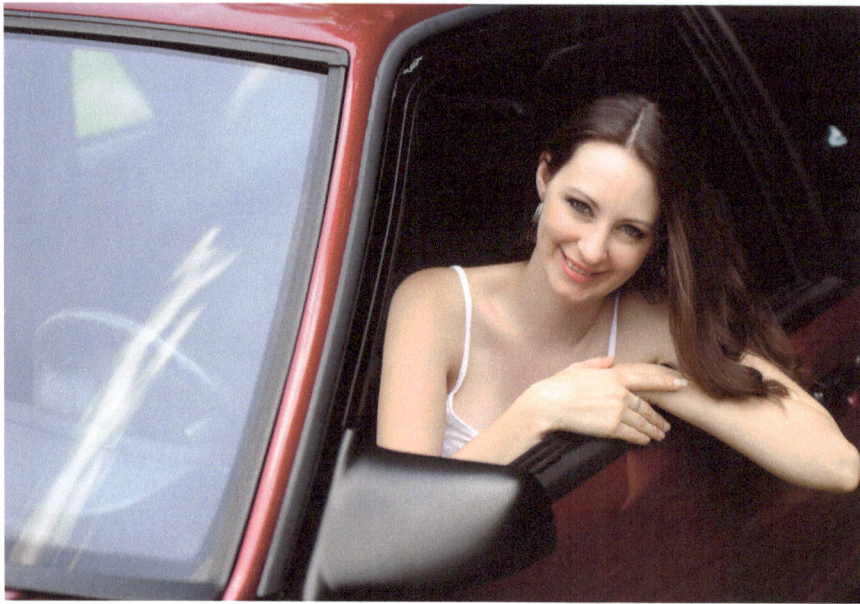

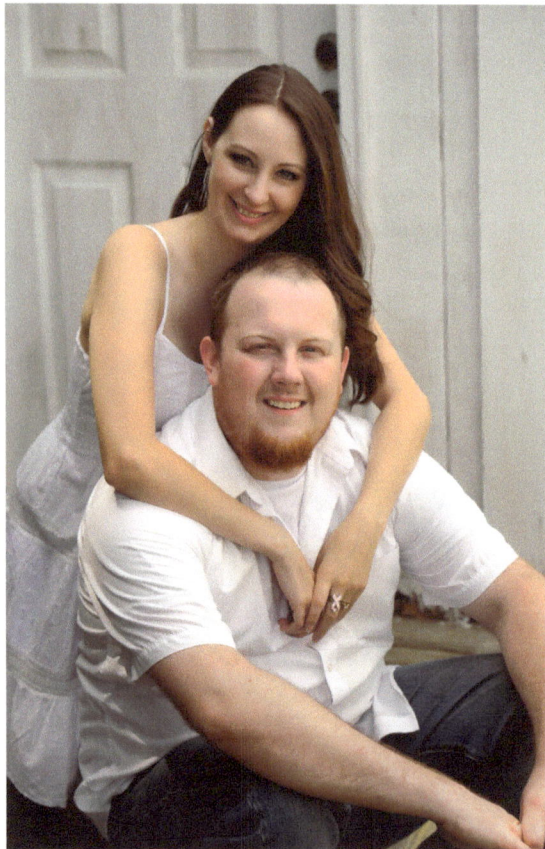

On May 7th, 2009, I had my mastectomy. I wanted them to take both breasts but because I was pregnant and had cancer in my lymph nodes, they didn't want me to be under anesthesia for that long.

On June 2nd, 2009 I had my first round of chemo. My pregnancy was going great and my baby girl was doing wonderful tolerating everything! My breast cancer was HER2 positive and hormone receptor positive. When the chemo treatments were over, I would start a year round antibody treatment every three weeks called "Herceptin".

On August 28, 2009, my miracle baby, Kennedy Hope Davis, was born. She was small but perfect. She stayed in the NICU for ten days.

I finished treatments in November and ended up getting a blood clot from my port. During emergency surgery, my port was removed. I started on blood thinners. This was frustrating, because I wanted to have reconstructive surgery so bad. I was getting so tired of only having one breast. I really wanted the other breast off as well! Being on blood thinners delayed the process.

Finally, in 2011, I visited my plastic surgeon. I was so excited at the thought of feeling normal again. It had been two and a half years since I had worn a pretty shirt or felt good about myself.

On May 13, I had my reconstructive surgery. I had my right breast removed and reconstructed at the same time. That helped relieve my worries of the cancer coming back in the right breast! After the expanders and healing time, it was time for the finaliza-

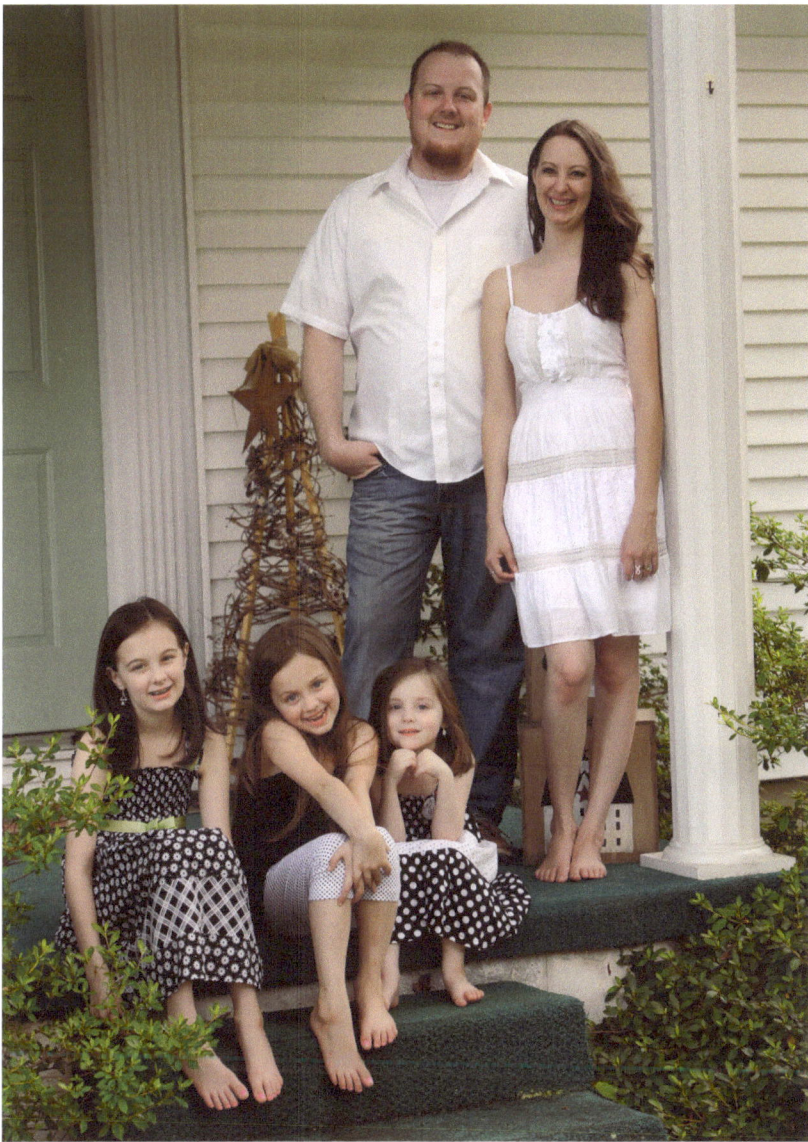

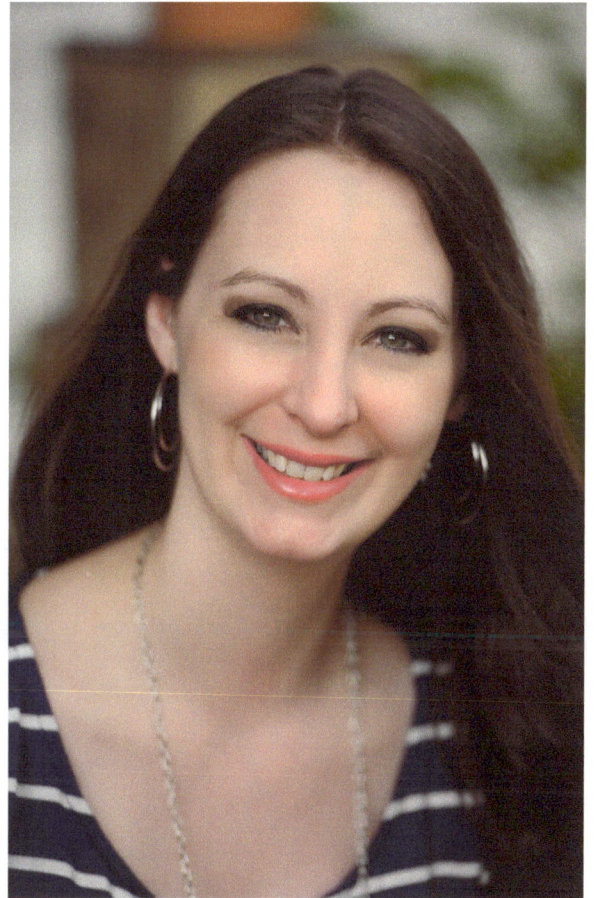

tion.

     I can't even express the feeling of having MY breasts back. I feel like a woman again! I can swim with my girls and just feel normal. I am so grateful for all my experiences, good and bad for they have made me the person I am today: A thankful, grateful person who lives everyday praising God for bringing me through and giving me the chance to raise my three beautiful girls.

     I am BLESSED!

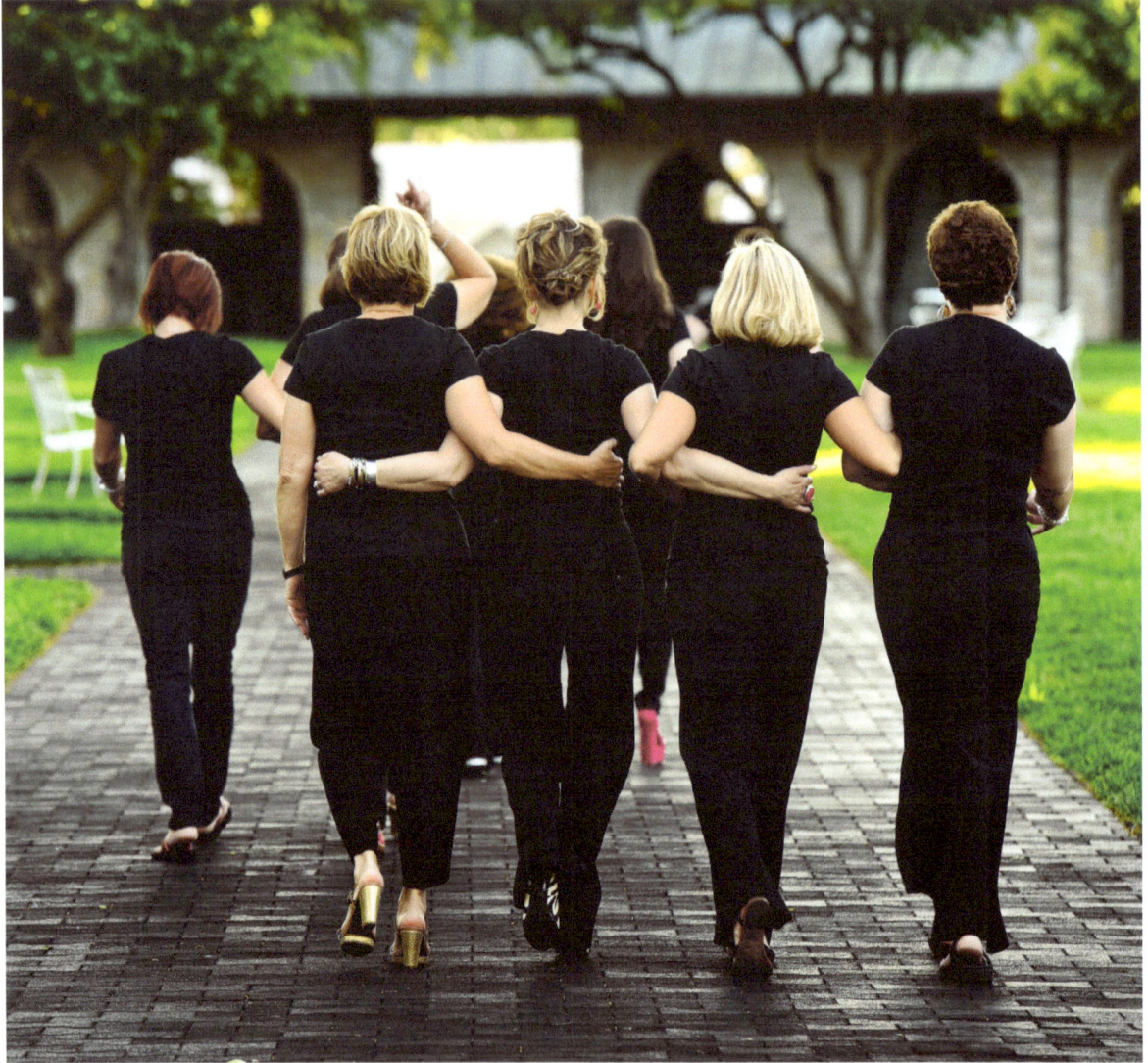

Pearls

There are numerous acceptable methods for reconstructing a breast—from an implant reconstruction at the time of the first surgical treatment to the complex operations involving flaps. All methods of breast reconstruction can be equally rewarding to the patient and the physician alike. In reconstructing a breast, there is no single technique that is suitable to all women. It takes careful consideration of all factors involved before choosing what could be a life changing decision.

I would like to share some "pearls" of wisdom that I have learned along the way in my practice to successfully reconstruct a breast with minimal "downtime" to the patient. This section is intended for physicians who diagnose and treat breast cancer, however, I have tried to keep the language as simple as possible, so if you have been diagnosed or you know of someone who has been diagnosed with breast cancer you will have some knowledge of how and why I choose a particular method for breast reconstruction. Please remember that each person diagnosed with breast cancer is unique and there is no single technique to reconstruct a breast that is suitable for all women.

The journey begins when a woman is first diagnosed with breast cancer. If the patient is a surgical candidate, evaluative appointments are scheduled with both a surgical oncologist and a plastic surgeon specializing in breast reconstruction. While the surgical oncologist is responsible for eliminating the cancer, the plastic surgeon is part of the "breast cancer team" to design the surgical incisions, which will result in a more aesthetically pleasing breast with minimal and well-hidden scars. In other words, the plastic surgeon is the "artist" who ensures the best possible cosmetic result.

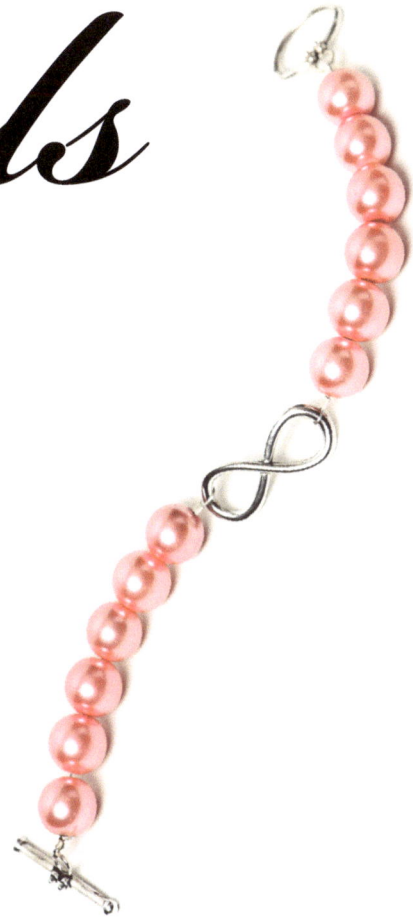

"New techniques for reconstructive surgery continue to evolve."

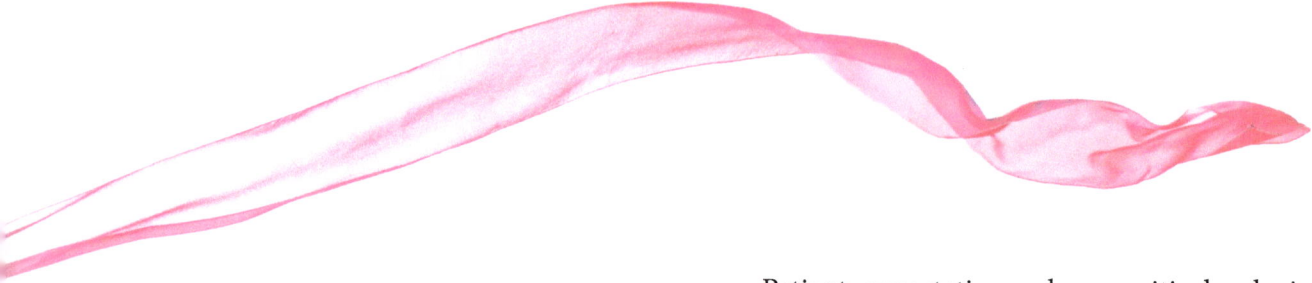

Patient expectations play a critical role in early surgical decision making. Does the patient want the easiest technique with the least amount of downtime for breast reconstruction—an implant—or does she want reconstruction with her own tissues? What is her age? What other health issues does she have? Is she obese, a smoker, had previous chest or abdominal surgery, or received radiation to the chest wall? These are just some very important questions that must be addressed before any type of breast surgery is planned.

New techniques for reconstructive surgery continue to evolve. FDA-approved breast implants are better tolerated by the body, and women are becoming more proactive in desiring to maintain their body image. With the advent of BRCA-1 gene testing for high-risk patients, more women are considering prophylactic mastectomies (e.g., Angelina Jolie) because they know they can be surgically reconstructed and look good without the worries of future breast cancer. Women are realizing that mastectomy may offer a higher chance for cure, and reconstruction can result in better aesthetics than conservation through a lumpectomy.

Every patient is unique. There are no magic numbers or designs, and there is no set protocol that is right for every woman. Women's breasts are different in size, shape, position, and skin type. Many factors affect breast reconstruction. For instance, in which quadrant of the breast is the cancer located? How deep to the overlying skin is it found? What is the tumor's relationship to the nipple areola complex? Are the breasts sagging, and how much excessive skin is there? How thick/thin is the skin?

A preoperative MRI is an extremely helpful test to diagnose where the cancer is located in the breast. The MRI is also helpful in analyzing skin thickness and location of the predominant blood supply to the breast.[1,5] which is information that is important to both the oncologic and reconstructive breast surgeon. Can the cancer surgeon safely preserve the blood supply to the skin without compromising the cancer removal? How thick is the skin? These are some questions that are answered while designing a mastectomy and reconstruction of the breast. Cancer and reconstructive plastic surgeons work together to offer a surgical cure while also maintaining aesthetic results. Whether performing a lumpectomy or mastectomy, collaboration offers the best possible outcome to the patient.

Preserve the Skin Envelope

For me, the key to aesthetic breast reconstruction is to preserve as much of the natural skin envelope of the breast as possible. Whether the patient desires a lumpectomy or a mastectomy, preservation of the overlying skin as long as the cancer is not invading the skin, is of utmost importance. While extra skin can be removed later, it is much more difficult to replace from the outset.
In patients with small, non-sagging breasts, the entire skin envelope is preserved. Skin-sparing mastectomies have become very popular, and a simple implant can make the breast look aesthetically better than it did before surgery. Either an incision in the inframammary fold or from the areola to the inframammary fold is all that is typically required. This vertical incision is usually not seen by the patient, as the majority of the scar is on the undersur-

"Skin-sparing mastectomies have become very popular"

face of the breast. In addition, this incision allows easier access to the axilla for the oncologic surgeon, should a lymph node biopsy be required. If a "lift" is desirable it can also be accomplished at the same time through this same vertical incision to provide a nice cosmetic result.

Removal of the nipple/areola is controversial but is the decision of the oncologic surgeon. Recent studies have shown that skin-sparing mastectomies can be oncologically safe with certain tumors and do not increase the risk of recurrence, especially if they are at least two centimeters from the nipple. However, if the nipple is flat and has little to no color, then there is little point in preservation. Nipple areola reconstruction might actually be more aesthetically pleasing. On the other hand, if there is a high projecting nipple and dark areolar skin that is of the appropriate diameter, saving the nipple areola can provide a more natural result. Even saving the areola while excising the central nipple leads to superior cosmetic results.

Of those patients who have minimal to moderate sagging, I would also attempt to save all of the skin. Fewer incisions lessen the risk of losing skin. Excess skin can be removed later if necessary. There is no point in compromising blood supply to the skin by adding more incisions during the first operation. The whole purpose of skin preservation is to maintain projection of the breast. The traditional mastectomy scar across the chest compromises projection of the breast and is not only visible to the patient looking down, but can be difficult to hide in clothing as well. Even with the most projecting implant available on the market today, a more aesthetically pleasing result can be obtained when incisions

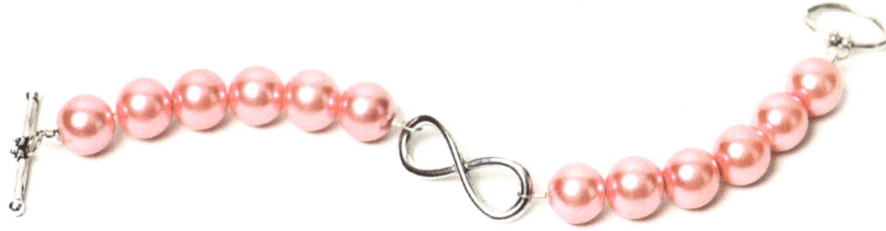

are created in the lower portion of the breast.

Mastopexy incisions—breast-lift techniques—should be avoided during the initial mastectomy in order to avoid compromising blood supply to the skin. Mastopexy incisions can be added once the initial trauma to the breast is healed. Immediate breast reconstruction at the time of a mastectomy makes it difficult to assess the viability of the skin in the operating room, so fewer incisions will lessen the risk of losing skin viability. Mastopexy incisions should only be considered if conservation breast surgery is planned, and the patient desires a breast lift.

For patients who have large, sagging breasts where the nipple is located far below the inframammary fold, removing excessive skin may be necessary but must be performed with caution. Breast reduction (Wise pattern) incisions can easily compromise the blood supply to the skin, especially if the skin flaps are very thin. When necessary, however, careful planning will allow the removal of excessive skin with little risk. Attention must be given to leaving intact all of the blood supply coming in from the sternum to the breast skin. Nipple-sparing mastectomies on large breasts can result in a viable nipple areola, which can be lifted at a later date if the blood supply coming from the sternum is not disturbed. If the blood supply to the nipple areola is in question, it is best to remove the nipple areola and "bank" it as a full thickness skin graft, to be transferred at a later time to the appropriate site.

"The whole purpose of saving skin is to save projection of the breast."

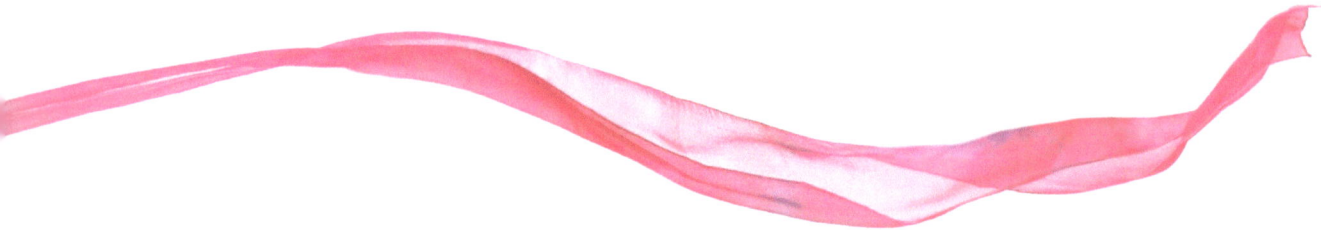

Breast Conservation Surgery

Plastic surgeons also should design the incisions when a patient desires breast conservation surgery. In patients with small breasts, the decision to perform a lumpectomy depends on the size of the tumor. If the tumor is so large that the cosmetic result is compromised as a result of the lumpectomy, a skin-sparing mastectomy may be a better option. The added effects of radiation therapy if a lumpectomy is performed will only worsen the cosmetic result and make reconstruction more challenging. On the other hand, if the breast is extremely large, it is helpful to design the lumpectomy as a breast reduction to help lessen the radiation dose required. The cosmetic result is also thus improved. A lumpectomy should not only save breast tissue, it should result in a cosmetically appealing breast—otherwise, there is no point since these patients are also irradiated. Irradiated breast tissue increases the risk of complications of breast reconstruction, so if a breast conservation surgery is desired, the results needs to look good from the start thus making breast reconstruction unnecessary.

Implant Breast Reconstruction

I have found that using breast implants to reconstruct a breast gives excellent results with minimal added time in the operating room and minimal added recovery time. Again, the new FDA approved breast implants gives excellent cosmetic results with fewer complications than were seen in the past. The size of the tissue expander is chosen based on the width and height of the breast. The tissue expander is placed below the muscle and inflated only to the point where there is no tension on the skin closure.

If the overlying skin is thin but shows good viability, it is preferable to use some form of human acellular dermis (treated cadaver skin). Acellular dermis is designed as an ellipse to fit into the lower outer quadrant of the breast and is attached to the chest wall at the level of the inframammary fold, as well as the border of the pectoralis major muscle above. This dermis allows proper placement of the tissue expander and adds protection and support to the expander, as well. Acellular dermis also helps thicken the skin to avoid the feel of the underlying implant. The tissue expander is then inflated on a weekly basis, typically two to three times, until the desired size is obtained.

I traditionally wait three months before changing the expander to a permanent implant, at which time additional revisions to the overlying skin can be made. Waiting three months allows the tissues enough time to heal and swelling to subside to obtain a more stable permanent result. Between operations, the patient may also receive chemotherapy if necessary.

In terms of breast implants, I have found that a smooth, round, gel implant with the highest projection gives an excellent aesthetic result. The newer form stable implants recently approved by the FDA also help provide an excellent aesthetic result for breast reconstruction.

It is sometimes necessary to revise the reconstruction later when the swelling has subsided—usually one year postoperatively. Often, there is lack of soft tissue relative to the implant in the upper pole of the breast, or there may be visible rippling from the under-

"FDA approved breast implants give an excellent cosmetic result with fewer complications than were seen in the past."

"My personal choice, if available, is the latissimus dorsi muscle."

lying implant because of thin skin flaps. Revising the breast reconstruction with the patient's own fat is a reliable and safe method to improve the result. The fat is liposuctioned into a sterile canister and then re-injected into the desired areas around the breast. The added soft tissue also improves the "feel" of the breast—making the breast feel more natural.

Flap Breast Reconstruction

Occasionally, the use of skin and muscle flaps may be necessary to reconstruct a breast. Skin and distant muscle flaps should only be used in breast reconstruction if an implant is not feasible, such as in cases where radiation was performed subsequent to a mastectomy and an additional source of blood supply is required. Using a breast implant alone in patients who have been radiated to the chest wall can be difficult and lead to many postoperative complications impossible to treat successfully.

If an implant breast reconstruction fails or is not possible, then flap reconstruction options such as the latissimus dorsi or TRAM (Transverse Rectus Abdominus Myocutaneous) flap as well as "free" flaps are available. The additional blood supply that these flaps provide allows reconstructing radiated tissue more feasible. My personal choice, if available, is the latissimus dorsi muscle. This flap provides a reliable blood supply and the procedure can be readily performed as an outpatient procedure with minimal downtime. This flap reconstructive option requires an implant to reconstruct the breast, but with the additional blood supply this flap provides, I have found that patients heal very nicely with excellent shape.

Conclusion

The whole point of an immediate breast reconstruction is that it allows the mastectomy patient to forget the fact they ever had breast cancer from the first time they were surgically treated. Breast reconstruction offers women with breast cancer something to look forward to. It gives them a sense of normalcy. They do not have the worry of a prosthesis falling out of their clothes, or have a caved-in looking chest. These women can still wear an evening gown or a bathing suit and feel good about it. They may even feel so good; they'd be willing to be photographed without their tops on. Best of all, if they end up looking better post-operatively than they did pre-operatively, well, then it's a home run, and it makes everyone involved feel great.

Life is too short not to enjoy every minute of every day. The key to treating breast cancer is early diagnosis and, if caught carly, you do not have to lose your breasts. Do not delay in getting a mammogram. Be proactive and seek help early. If you have recently been diagnosed with breast cancer or if you are a physician who treats patients with breast cancer, make sure you have a plastic surgeon involved from the time of diagnosis. You will be glad you did.

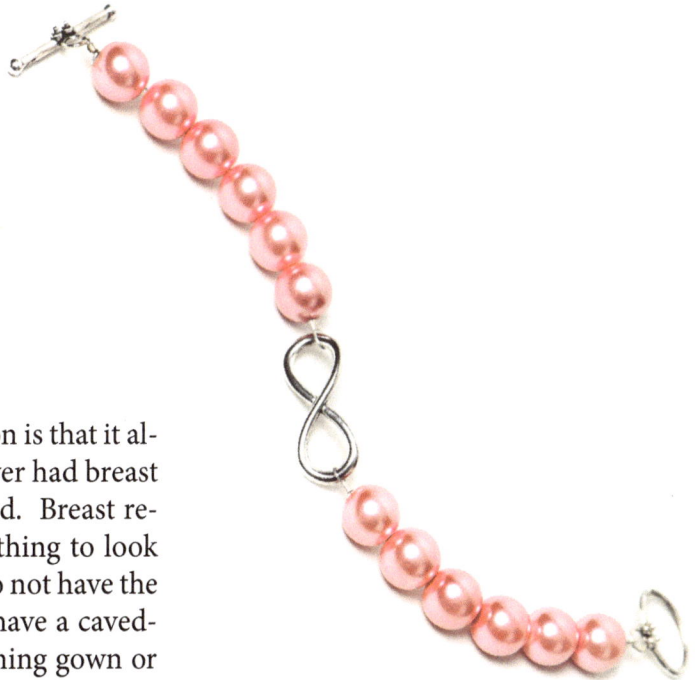

Vision

Scott Walz, M. Photog, Cr.

Awe inspiring courage. That is a fraction of the respect I hope for all of the ladies involved and portrayed in this book. When Dr. Bouzaglou asked me to be involved in this project in December of 2012 I was open to the idea because of my personal experiences with breast cancer. Thirty years ago, when I was 19 and my sister Carole was 32, we got the news that she had breast cancer. It didn't seem real and at the time I was sure she would survive. Unfortunately I was wrong and she went through an ordeal of surgeries, radiation treatments and punishing chemotherapies. Sadly, she passed away after five years of fighting for her life.

I have also had a long list of friends and family members that have had to deal with the pain of breast cancer so I really wanted to help where I could. This, however, was a new twist to me when considering surviving breast cancer. So much information is out there encouraging women to do self-exams and to get regular mammograms and I had become familiar with the terms "lumpectomy", "mastectomy" and "bi-lateral mastectomy" I really had never thought much about breast reconstruction and how it worked.

The thought of photographing women who had beaten cancer and who wanted to feel whole again was exciting. The thought of photographing them topless scared me to death. I didn't want the images to change people's opinions about our studio but after long consideration I agreed to work on the project. If one woman could be helped to find happiness again after surviving breast cancer through images lovingly created then I felt that I had to step up and do my best.

Then life threw in one of those twists that shake you to your core. In January, just a month after agreeing to help with this book, my darling wife was diagnosed with breast cancer. We were now right in the midst of the struggle and decisions that faced all of the women in this book. I can't really know how they feel and what they have really gone through just as I can't really know what Valorie, my wife, has really suffered.

I can however, testify to the strength, courage, inner and outer beauty of Valorie and these ladies. This book is a love song to all of them. Those of you who have the great privilege to call these women wife, mother, sister and daughter know how I feel. If they had not had breast reconstruction they would still be beautiful, incredible women but they chose to own their bodies and their beauty and all I can do is be humbled and in awe of them.

I miss my sister Carole terribly but I thank God for my incredible wife. Valorie I love you and think you are and always have been the most beautiful woman in the world.

Thank You

I want to first thank each of these wonderful ladies for agreeing to participate in this book project. Though we met through their illness, I feel blessed that our paths have crossed. They have made me realize how important life is and why I have been doing what I do for so long. Together with them, I am hoping this project will make a difference in how women perceive breast cancer throughout the world.

Every so often in life we get to meet people who make a positive difference to everyone around them. Genea Arrasmith, is one of them. She has been the guiding force behind this entire group. Genea is, no doubt, the most positive breast cancer survivor Kentucky has ever seen and for this I have given her the title of "Kentucky's Patient Courage, 2013". As the tattoo that she bears on her wrist states, "NO FEAR", she truly has no fear. I love her dearly and look up to her for her positive energy and smile. Best of all, she has become a true friend, not just to me, but to many other breast cancer survivors that she has come to know over the past several years.

I want to thank all of my staff throughout the years: Christie Aspden and Jeanne McGuire, who helped me start my practice more than twenty years ago, and then Denise Sparks, Samantha Shimfessel-Mastin, Marty Hall, Rewa Smith, Dr. Sandra Roberts, and all who have worked at the Center for Plastic Surgery and The SurgiCenter. I sincerely appreciate all of their hard work and dedication. I especially thank Denise for all of her volunteer hours towards this project going far beyond her job requirements. Her dedication to this project deserves special recognition.

I also thank my physicians assistant, Paige Hoogerheide, who has been on the opposite side of the operating table for the majority of the breast reconstructions I have performed over the past 10 years. She also designed and made the beautiful scarves that you see the ladies wearing throughout the book. She is a true artist and her assistance in the operating room is invaluable.

Thank you to our editor, Cynthia Ellingsen, for editing all of the amazing stories written by our patients themselves. She was so kind in offering her services to this important project.

Thank you, too, to our wonderful photographer, Scott Walz. He has been absolutely amazing in capturing the true spirit of each of our patients. I could not have done this project without him. He and his beautiful wife, Valorie, have become like family to me, and I love them both.

Last, I thank my magnificent husband, Sandy; my four children, Daniel, Joshua, Ethan and Dahlia; and my dear nanny, Heidi, for supporting me throughout my professional career. They understand all of the hard work that went into this project and how much it meant, not only to me but to these lovely ladies as well. I love you all.

Procedures

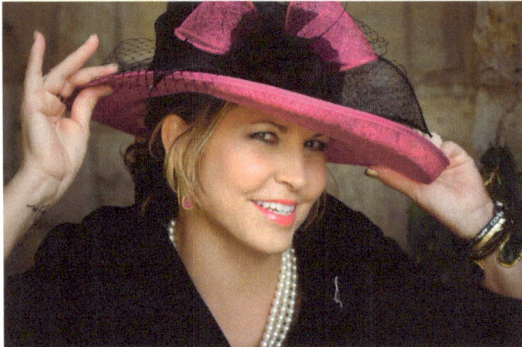

Genea: Right skin sparing mastectomy, Left mastectomy with immediate breast reconstruction (designed incisions) with tissue expanders followed by permanent gel implants

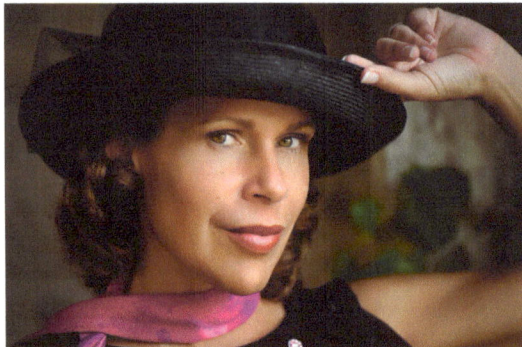

Alycia: Right mastectomy (designed incisions) with immediate breast reconstruction with tissue expanders followed by permanent implant; Left augmentation mastopexy

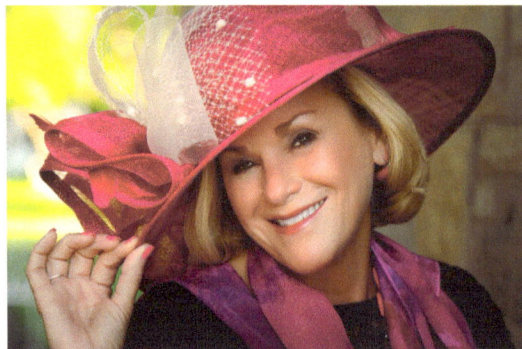

Sandy: Bilateral mastectomies (designed incisions) with immediate reconstruction tissue expander/permanent gel implant

Sherry: Bilateral mastectomies (designed incisions) with immediate breast reconstruction and tissue expander/permanent gel implants, tattooing of nipple areola

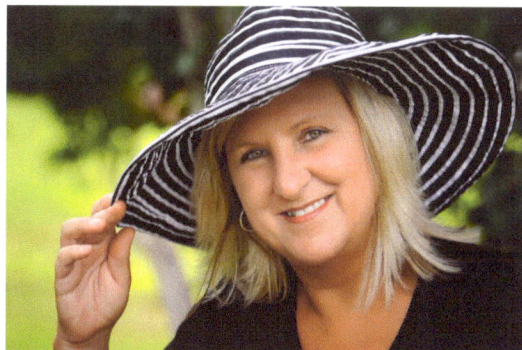

Beverly: Right lumpectomy with post-op radiation, delayed breast reconstruction with permanent gel implant, Left breast augmentation

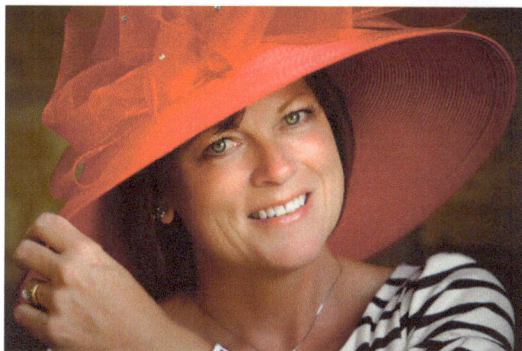

Jill: Bilateral mastectomies (designed incisions) with immediate breast reconstruction tissue expander/permanent gel implant

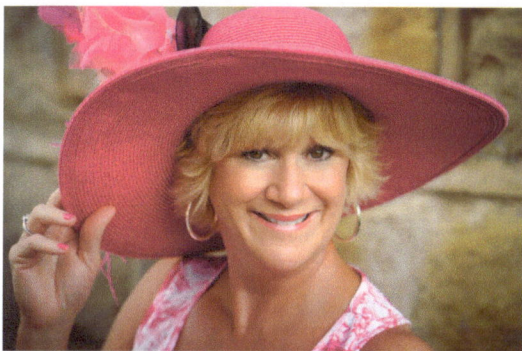

Mary: Left mastectomy (designed incisions) with immediate breast reconstruction with tissue expanders, Right augmentation mastopexy

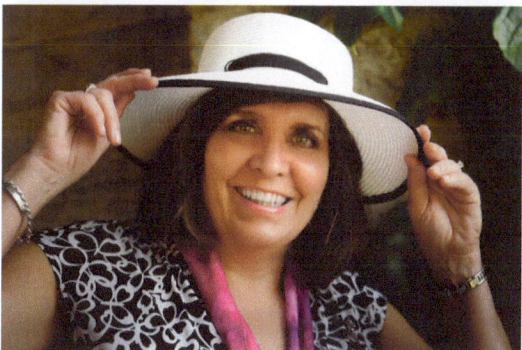

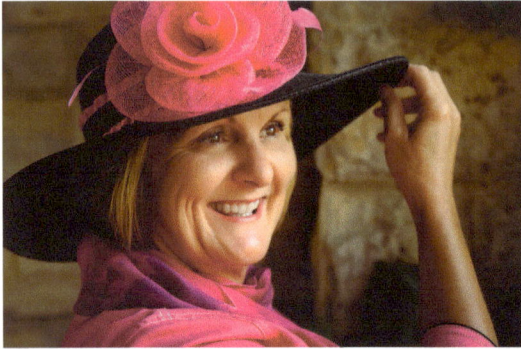

Lisa : Bilateral breast reduction followed by bilateral mastectomies (using Wise pattern incisions) with immediate tissue expander breast reconstruction with nipple areolar banking and subsequent permanent implant and nipple reconstruction with banked nipple and tattoo of areola

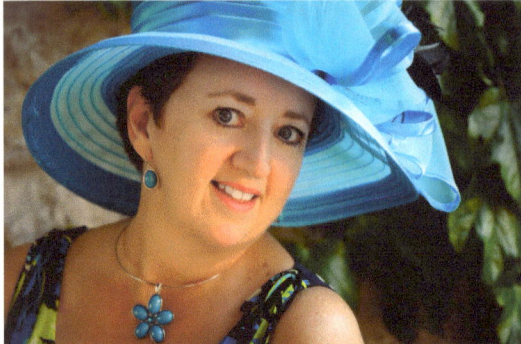

Susan: Bilateral mastectomies (designed incisions) with immediate tissue expander reconstruction

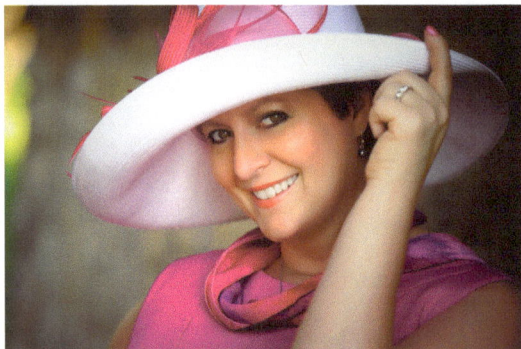

Lisa: Bilateral mastectomies with delayed tissue expander breast reconstruction with mastopexy incisions to remove excess skin, permanent gel implant

Shawna: Right lumpectomy and radiation, followed by right mastectomy and left skin sparing mastectomy (designed incisions) with immediate tissue expander breast reconstruction and subsequent permanent implant and a delayed mastopexy on the left side

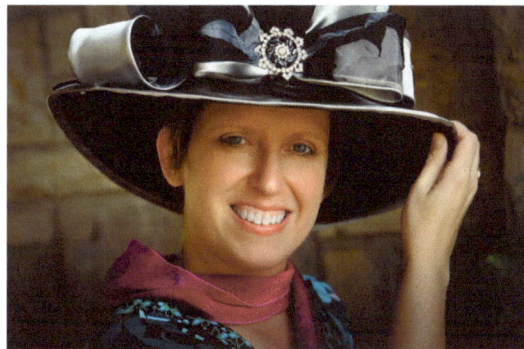

Marsha: Right mastectomy and delayed expander breast reconstruction. Left mastectomy (designed incisions) with immediate expander breast reconstruction followed by bilateral permanent gel implants

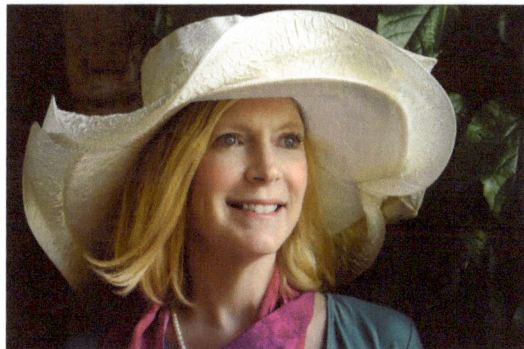

Holly: Left Mastectomy followed by delayed expander breast reconstruction. Right mastectomy (incisions designed) with immediate expander breast reconstruction followed by permanent gel implant breast reconstruction. Tattooing of nipple areolae

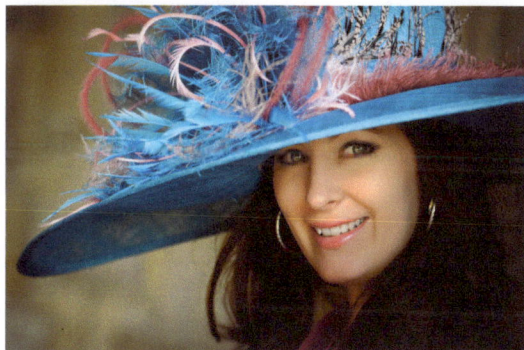

References

1. De Angelis R, Tavilla A, Verdecchia A, et al. Breast cancer survivors in the United States: Geographic variability and time trends, 2005-2015. Cancer 2009;1954-1966

2. Wang HT,Barone CM,Steigelman MB,et al. Aesthetic outcomes in breast conservation therapy. Aesthet Surg J. 2010;28:165-170.

3. Soltanian H,Okada H. Understanding genetic analysis for breast cancer and its implications for plastic surgery. Aesthet Surg J. 2010;28:85-91

4. Alderman AK,McMahon L Jr, Wilkins EG. The national utilization of immediate and early delayed breast reconstruction and the effect of sociodemographic factors. Plastic Reconstr Surg. 2003:111:695-703;discussion 704-705

5. Seitz,Iris A.MD,PhD; Friedwald,Sarah MD; et al Breast MRI Helps Define the Blood Supply to the Nipple-Areolar Complex. Plastic & Reconst Surg: October 2010-Vol 126 Issue-p 27

6. Alderman AK,HawleyST, Waljee J, et al. Correlates of referral practices of general surgeons to plastic surgeons for mastectomy reconstruction. Cancer 2007;109:1715-1720

7. Garfein,ES, MD. The Privilege of Advocacy:Legislating Awareness of Breast Reconstruction, Plastic Reconstr Surg J. Sept 2011

8. Serletti,J MD, Fosnot,J,MD et al Breast Reconstruction after Breast Cancer. Plast Recons Surg June 2011-Vol 127-Issue pp124e-135e

9. American Society of Plastic Surgeons "Breast Cancer Patient Education Act" ,www.plasticsurgery.org

Resources

www.cancer.org
www.plasticsurgery.org
www.bcaction.org
www.Breastcancer.org
www.breastimplantanswers.com/
www.Natrelle.com
www.mentorwwllc.com
www.kypinkconnection.com
www.center4plasticsurgery.com
www.komen.org

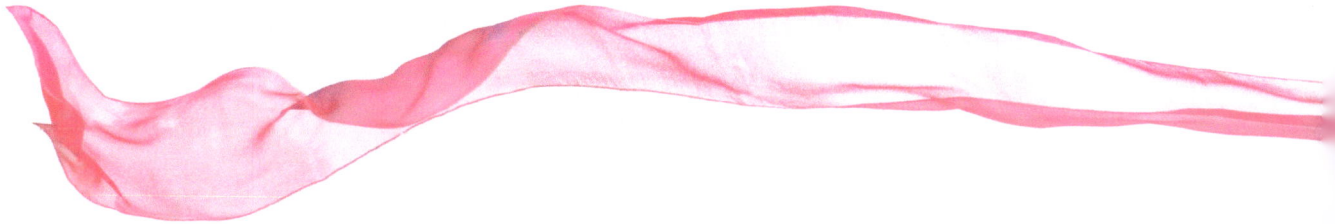

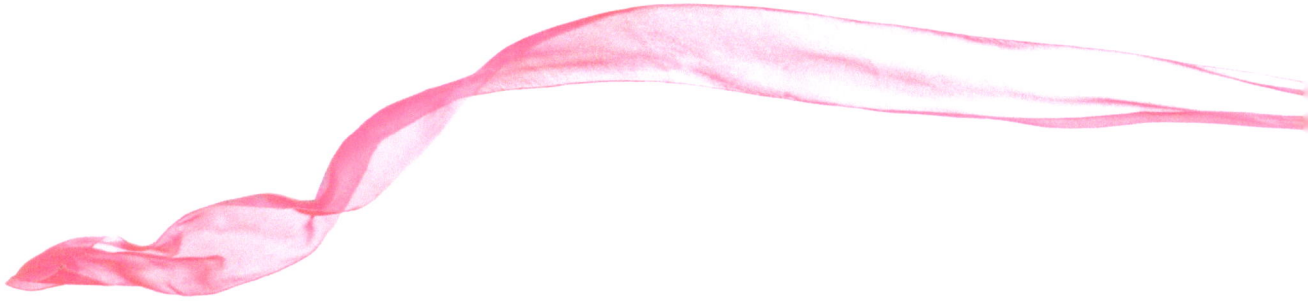

Sandra Bouzaglou, MD FACS, is a plastic surgeon living in Lexington, Kentucky. After undergraduate training at UCLA, she graduated from The Chicago Medical School, then completed five years of general surgery at The University of Iowa and a Plastic Surgery Fellowship at The University of Kentucky. She is the founder of The Center for Plastic Surgery and The SurgiCenter, Kentucky's first AAAASF outpatient surgical facility in Lexington, Kentucky.

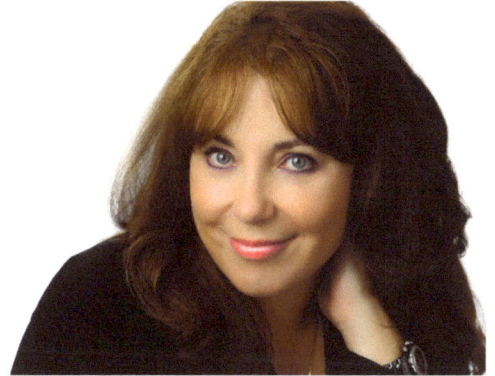

Scott Walz is a Lexington, Kentucky based photographer who began working professionally at the age of sixteen. In college he initially majored in engineering but eventually succumbed to his joy of photography. The study of physics and optics and combined well with his study of art and design. Scott and his wife Valorie established their own business in Lexington in 1992 and since then Studio Walz, Inc. has grown steadily and they are grateful for the support of their many loyal customers.

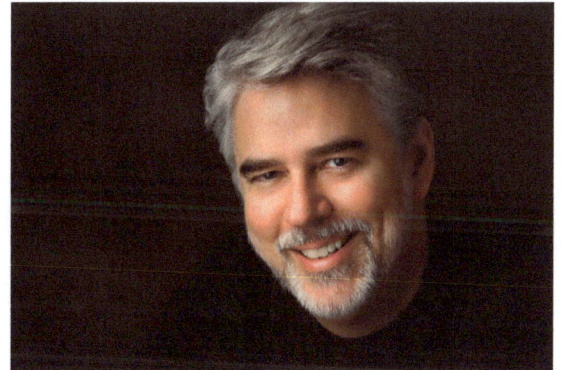

www.ingramcontent.com/pod-product-compliance
Lightning Source LLC
Chambersburg PA
CBHW041448210326
41599CB00004B/171